Finding Serenity

*How Yoga and Positive Self-Talk
Can Take you from
Not-My-Day to Namaste*

"Let go of your story so the universe can write
you a new one."

Marianne Williamson

Table of Contents

Introduction

I started practicing yoga many, many years ago. I must admit that the first time I attended a class was not very inspirational and it is a wonder that I continued. It was in an austere, two-storey building in the downtown core. Paint peeled from the walls, the windows were dirty, and the floor was as cold as the atmosphere. But, being the good people-pleaser that I was, and can still be today, I persevered and smiled reverently at the teacher. For me, people pleasing was a coping strategy and that had become a deeply entrenched behavior. Trauma, which began in childhood, had left me feeling afraid most of the time. During the class, I worried if what I had on was appropriate and spiritual enough. I didn't have a yoga mat so I brought a towel, as the flyer suggested. I tried to do the poses in a competent manner. I finished the class, even though I was cold and could hardly hear the teacher from the back, which I had chosen to avoid being seen.

I felt awkward and out of place, but I sensed that yoga was good for me. Little did I know that, years later, I would become a yoga teacher. Perhaps I understood that there were benefits beyond becoming more "stretchy"; I sensed that it was good for my mind as well as my body.

The teacher concentrated on the breath. Much later, I realized that the shallow breathing I had engaged in everyday of my life was an effort to quash my emotions: positive, negative, somewhat loving, or hateful. That was also when I realized that fearful, negative thoughts were dominating my life.

Something kept bringing me back to yoga and I returned to it sporadically over many years. Intuitively, I knew that yoga helped me to deal with my negative self-talk, which I projected onto others and the world. My negativity made the world uncomfortable and unsafe, but I felt a little less fearful and a little more peaceful after I finished a class. There were times when my constant, anxious self-talk would cease and my mind would go quiet. For a few moments I would feel "normal," rather than the worst person in the world. So, I kept at it.

Over time, I noticed recurring themes in the thoughts running through my mind. They were rooted in feelings of unworthiness and insecurity. It took many more years of therapy and yoga to uncover the core beliefs that had led to those feelings: I didn't deserve to be happy; I was not good enough, and, most importantly, the world was *a scary place*. Years later, I would become a therapist myself; committed to helping others become more resilient through personal growth.

Early in my journey, yoga helped me recognize the dominant thought patterns that were making me feel so terrible about myself. Was it possible to change how I felt? Could I find a person inside my own body that I could love and feel content with? One that could make mistakes without experiencing the sharp, piercing pangs of shame and self-loathing?

I doubt I was consciously aware that I was even thinking these deep, life-altering thoughts at the time. I was too busy trying to live in a scary world of my own making. I told myself it would get better one day and that eventually the panic attacks would stop.

Meanwhile, I would spend some days gasping for air constantly, resorting to very shallow breathing to conserve energy.

I felt like such a fake; a phoney pretending that I was a happy, go-lucky person. I was trying to appear successful. I wanted people to believe that I had my shit together, that I was happy. Far from it. When I got older, I realized that the panic attacks and the use of alcohol to self-soothe were signs that, deep down inside, I was living a lie.

I had a pretty good life: I had a good job, a wonderful partner, and an instant family that I was grateful for despite the challenges of being a stepparent. What I didn't know at the time, was that my continued practice of yoga and increasing "stretchiness" would eventually expose an area of my life in desperate need of fixing.

Yoga allowed my dark, negative thoughts about myself to surface more often, which increased my anxiety levels. I couldn't keep them out, particularly when I was relaxing in Shavasana, or final relaxation.

I noticed that the lie I was living was more apparent when I focused on my "go-to" thoughts and attitudes about myself. I knew I needed something to help me work on my mind and constant negativity.

My go-to thoughts, and the core beliefs they reflected, simply *sucked!* They were dark and foreboding. They reminded me continually that I was defective; that I was less than, and separate from, everyone else. They told me that everyone hated me and was out to get me. Sometimes they shouted that no one really liked me, that I was incompetent, and that I therefore had to be *ultra-nice* and *super-helpful* in order to make up for my huge, glaring faults.

I became even more of a people-pleaser: I would dress a certain way, talk a certain way, *live* a certain way, so as not to rock the boat. I thought that maybe, if I could just be agreeable and tell people what they wanted to hear, I could be somewhat accepted.

As you can imagine, the constant influence of my negative core beliefs on my thinking, was terrifying and embarrassing. I was supposed to have it all together, so, in response, I doubled-down on looking perfect, trying harder at my job, and working harder on perfecting my effervescent façade.

But, what goes up must come down and, inevitably, I crashed in a big way. After hitting rock-bottom, I finally decided to join a 12-step support group and began practising real self-improvement.

As I worked on forgiving myself and practising self-acceptance for my real or imagined faults, I discovered that if I wanted to develop lasting self-acceptance and awareness, I needed to do more than just attend yoga classes and do the poses. It required constant vigilance to keep those familiar, judgmental thoughts about myself out of my head, and to control my thoughts in a heart-centered, loving way. It was transformational.

Once I realized that my unhealthy beliefs were trying to protect me by suppressing childhood memories of the trauma I experienced as a witness to violence in my home, I began to heal. It is an on-going process but I am living proof that there is light at the end of that judgemental, self-critical tunnel.

I wrote this book to share what I have learned along the way and help others navigate through trauma to joy. I have purposely chosen not to detail the events that led to my own trauma, in part to protect myself, but also to avoid triggering traumatic memories in my readers. Instead I have focused on the recovery process and lessons learned along the way. Even if you have not experienced trauma yourself, I believe that anyone struggling with anxiety or depression will benefit from its content.

In the following chapters, I discuss what Cognitive Behavioural Therapists call Cognitive Distortions. I talk about my feelings of perfectionism, over-personalisation, self-criticism, and judgement. I describe what it is like to feel separate and alone and how I used impression management to prevent others from thinking that I was a terrible person.

I recount how I climbed out of the pit of self-criticism and fear through a process of acceptance, forgiveness, allowing for mistakes to be made, being real, and self-care. Each step in the process has helped me land on the happier, sunny shores of my interior landscape that were just waiting to be discovered and enjoyed. For me, it was yoga and a stillness practice that helped me tap into those happier places. They still do.

Practicing yoga and monitoring my thoughts using Cognitive Behavioural Therapy (CBT) techniques, really accelerated my healing process. Yoga helped heal my body and CBT, infused with love, helped heal my mind. I accept myself now. When I teach yoga, I start by describing myself as imperfect. It is good medicine, a good reminder that no one is perfect, including me.

My glass is half-full now, the positive far outweighing the negative, which is why, although I do use my experience for illustrative purposes, the vast majority of this book is about solutions not problems. It is an imperfect yogini's story about cultivating the inner witness through yoga and mindfulness. I hope you enjoy it.

I went from "Not My Day, to Namaste." Now I want to help you get there too.

Holly

Part 1:

Problematic Thinking

The wound is the place

where the Light enters in.

Rumi.

Chapter 1:
Perfectionism

Ego Mantra: I will never be acceptable as I am.

vs

Heart Mantra: I unconditionally accept myself.

Wisdom from Yoga and Getting Quiet:

Being in the moment and accepting whatever we are feeling emotionally and physically helps to identify whatever it is we need to feel. Our bodies never lie. Being with whatever is surfacing helps painful emotional and physical feelings to pass. They stop chasing us to get our attention.

Why is everyone perfect and I'm not?

The first time I consciously believed that I was not perfect while others were, was when I compared my family life to that of my best friend. I decided that everything about her family was not only very different from mine, it was also everything I wanted. Her house, parents, siblings, pets, were what I thought I should have in life. I also came to believe that if I tried hard enough and was a good girl, student, friend, and daughter, I could be accepted by her family, which would mean I was good enough and could possibly be perfect as well. Perfection was something to strive for. Much later, I understood that trying to be perfect distracted me from the conflict happening in my home. If I could hang out with my friend at school and at her home with her wonderful family, I could survive in life and be thought of as perfect too— reasoning that led to many, many years of worry, anxiety, and self-loathing.

This became the story I was invested in maintaining. I thought that if I could be like my friend or anyone in her family, I would be acceptable. Now, there is something to be said about having role models in your life, however, when these role models are "perfect" in your mind, and therefore not human, they cease to be realistic. We all know that perfection is unattainable. It is not humanly possible. We all screw up and fall short of the mark once in a while. Unfortunately for me, her family became my sole source of validation. If she and her family liked me, then I was likeable and perfect; if they didn't, I wasn't.

If they thought that I was smart because of how well I performed at school, I was okay. I was an A+ people-pleaser. I hadn't developed my own sense of worth, which is usually nurtured by our parents and teachers, so I constantly sought external validation. As it was, I don't remember caring if my parents or teachers liked me as much as I cared that her perfect family did.

Although I performed well academically, it didn't really matter to me. What I wanted was to be athletic like my friend and her siblings. Good grades were fine, but I sensed that her family valued physical prowess more. So, not only did I devalue what I was good at, I felt distant and alone much of the time because I did not measure up athletically. I was tall for my age and felt awkward compared to my friend who was shorter. My awkwardness held me back; I was too embarrassed to train to be better at athletics. Unbeknownst to me, negativity, and its domino effect, had already started to set in.

Instead of accepting that we all have different gifts and interests, I felt that I was lacking. I just couldn't match my friend's performance; I was not going to be perfect after all. I concluded that, since I was not good at swimming, running, or any track and field events for that matter, her family would notice that I was not perfect like their daughter was. Therefore, it would be impossible for them to like me. One negative thought led to another.

The problem with perfectionism and negativity is that they make us feel truly defective. We never measure up to the ridiculously high standards we set for ourselves. We feel unworthy and undeserving of happiness, of success, of peace, of *love*. Our minds are chaotic; we worry about not keeping up the appearance of perfection and therefore not really fitting in or being accepted. I wish I had realized that my feelings were not unusual. Many people, especially adolescents, feel insecure and suffer from anxiety. I thought that if I worked hard, never made any mistakes, and was super-nice, I could still fit into the ideal world that I had created in my mind of what life was supposed to be like; a world where everyone was perfect and never made any mistakes.

Another reason that seeking external validation sets us up for an emotional fall is your source of validation may disappear one day. This happened when my friend's family moved to the other side of town. Their validation of me was gone and, with it, my anchor, my safe harbour. I felt more fearful and had more anxiety attacks as my breathing became more and more unpredictable. The stress caused me to regularly break out in cold sores, which only increased my need to be perfect. I was entering high school and felt ugly.

Our body never lies. It sends signals that we should pay attention to. My shortness of breath, cold sores, and upset stomach were all warnings that I needed to heed. There was no amount of being nice or people pleasing that could take away the emotional pain I was experiencing. Terrible cold sores on my mouth deepened my self-loathing, and feelings of isolation. Smoking exacerbated the feeling. I knew cigarettes were not healthy, but I wanted to fit in. I was in a terrible bind and sinking fast without a lifeline to reach for. Except maybe for alcohol, which helped ease the pain.

Yoga: I am so glad yoga and mindfulness are now being taught in some schools. If we also add positive and loving self-talk to the curriculum, children will have a mental health practice they can do for life.

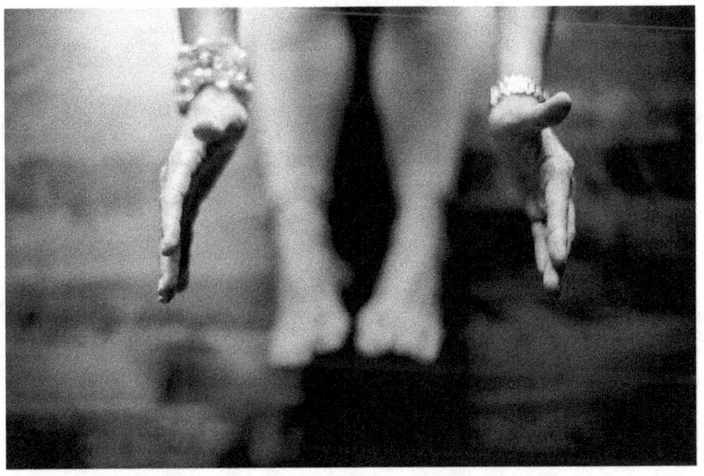

Yoga Pose: Holding the pose Sitting Forward Fold is all about going forward and embracing it. Holding it longer takes faith and trust.

Chapter 2

Over-Personalizing and Self-Criticism

> *Ego Mantra: I constantly compare*
> *myself to others.*
>
> *vs*
>
> *Heart Mantra: I accept that we*
> *all have unique gifts.*

Yoga and Meditation Wisdom:

If we get quiet and still enough, we can travel inward and find peace. We will tap into a luminous being that is waiting to emerge. But it takes a great deal of self-acceptance and Ego awareness.

Why do I hate myself so much?

During adolescence we wonder what people think of us. We all want to know that we matter, that we count. We want to know that people want to hang out with us. In my case, the constant, insecure self-talk made me think that everyone was thinking and talking negatively about me. I was on high alert for the slightest look of disapproval or disappointment. I over-personalized their every move and thought it was about *me*. Witnessing abuse when you are young can feel like you are the one being abused, so you don't want to upset or anger anyone. I believed that, if I was nice and did not rock the boat and agreed with everything you said, I would escape unscathed. I would be liked. I wouldn't get hurt.

Being constantly on-guard against any negativity directed toward me was exhausting. I realized much later that people were not thinking about me. They were thinking about themselves. They were wrapped-up in their own life, trying to live in the moment as best they could. Those around me were dealing with their own issues of insecurity or disappointment in their lives. The more fortunate ones would be accepting of whatever was happening and would deal with it. Even though I was an introvert for the most part, I spent much more time directing my thoughts and energy outwards rather than checking in with myself to see how I was feeling and behaving. Again, focusing on others helped me avoid the emotional pain I was in, which was a form of denial.

So, a typical hour in my head was similar to being an air-traffic controller. Regardless of how old I was or what job I was doing at the time, I would constantly be monitoring and on alert for incoming opinions about me. I would be assessing and re-assessing every second that someone was talking to me for signs of approval or disapproval. If their eyes or mouth twitched, I would become alarmed. I then had to decide whether or not they were going to hurt me somehow. They might say something to me that would make me feel incompetent or stupid, or they might make a negative comment about me to someone else. In the professional context, I worried that a person in power might hold back a promotion or fire me. Or, worst-case scenario, I wondered if the other person might physically harm me. These were my daily concerns. They were very real.

If I detected negative feed-back from someone, my only line of defense was to remain nice and totally agree with whatever they were saying, regardless of whether or not I felt their opinion was justified. Unfortunately, when you're trying to be "sugar and spice and everything nice", you lose your inner compass. Your sense of self depends totally on what others think and whether they like you. You stop checking in with yourself to see how you feel and what your truth is, if you ever checked in at all. When this occurs, a great deal of unconscious anger begins to build within you.

I once heard that depression was "anger turned inside." I have come to believe that there are many types and levels of depression, which range from having minor anxiety to completely shutting down. When we're depressed, we tend to retreat inside our shell for protection and try to self-soothe as best we can, which can take an enormous amount of energy. We now know that negative and depressive thoughts emit stress hormones that are not good for our bodies.

Neuroscience has also proven that after thinking so many negative thoughts, our mind begins to produce them automatically as it tries to anticipate danger and protect us from it. The result is: *fight, flight, freeze or appease.*

People who have experienced trauma, quite frequently believe that everything is unsafe. When I was researching domestic violence, I learned that men who feel threatened and unsafe often act-out by using violence and projecting a toughness, otherwise known as "fight". Many women, like myself, resort to people-pleasing, or "freeze or appease," behavior.

I would get cut off by another car and believe the driver was angry and out to get me. I would walk into a washroom at work and wonder if the women there were talking about me and stopped when they heard me enter. I projected the fear that I was feeling onto others and felt that they were unsafe to be around. I also wondered if they were thinking about me the same way I was thinking about myself, negatively and judgmentally.

I was so critical of myself and so afraid of failure that I didn't believe I was capable of succeeding in a post-secondary school. I had the choice between two academic paths. The first, was a shorter high school program, designed for students who wanted to attend college or enter the workforce immediately after graduation. The second, was for those interested in University. That option took a year longer. Although my elementary teacher had encouraged me to believe in myself and my academic ability, I chose the shorter program. My teacher had wanted me to attend university and to choose the most direct path to get there, even if it meant an extra year of high school. I was too critical of myself to trust his recommendation. My self-critic would not allow me to entertain the idea of taking the university aptitude test. Before leaving high school, I considered attending a community college and pursuing a career in law because I had achieved a very high mark in a related course. Thankfully, I started working instead; I would have made a terrible law clerk.

That self-criticism was yet another consequence of my perfectionism and triggered panic attacks. Not feeling good or perfect enough would start a stream of negative self-talk that would lead to an inevitably negative conclusion: why start something new, when I would only fail at it? Why try to make new friends, when they would not really like me anyway? Believing that I would be exposed and hurt in someway led to panic and affected every area of my life.

Shallow breathing and anxiety went hand in hand. I often could not breathe and gasped for air. In order to get a breath, I would visualize trying to climb up and over a mountain, where the air was fresh and I could breathe more easily. Sometimes it worked. Other times,

I just kept trying. Or, I would try yawning to get a full breath. Being unable to breathe because of the stress of the moment could easily trigger an anxiety attack.

My anxiety and panic were reflexive; they activated without my knowledge or control. Looking back, I am sure that they were automatic responses that masked and attempted to quash other emotions such as sadness and confusion. Alcohol helped me feel calmer, but it was a two-edged sword. Domestic violence workers know this and will often tell their clients not to, "over-do alcohol or drugs of any kind." Mind-altering substances make victims more susceptible to abuse by dulling the senses causing them to miss the warning signs of danger.

I felt alone most of the time because I was off cut-off from "real" connection. I enjoyed my friends as best I could and got as close to them as I was able, but there was still a degree of closeness that was missing. As I ventured out into the world because it was getting too difficult to hide my defects in my hometown, I began to gravitate toward people who did not have my best interests at heart.

People pleasers need more powerful people to appease. I was often using alcohol to self-soothe, so guess what kind of people I attracted? Yes, people with issues and something to prove. As the family violence workers had predicted, I found myself ignoring the warning signs and remaining in unhealthy relationships or situations for too long, which only confirmed that I was a defective person.

A wonderful person would be happy. A wonderful person would be self-confident, able to venture into the world without self-medicating and able to stay away from predators. I felt like a victim and, looking back now, I can see I was deliberately targeting people who made me feel that way. I was always on edge and would *freeze or appease* at the slightest hint of danger when I should have run the other way. Even if I was alone and out of harm's way, it seems that my brain was still scanning for dangerous situations and people. I later realized that the survival part my brain felt threatened and under siege most of the time, that is why it remained hyper-vigilant and over-anxious.

Yoga: Helped me become aware of my body and my feelings by sitting quietly with my eyes softly opened or closed. This helped to silence the outside world. Surprisingly, I felt safe and calm.

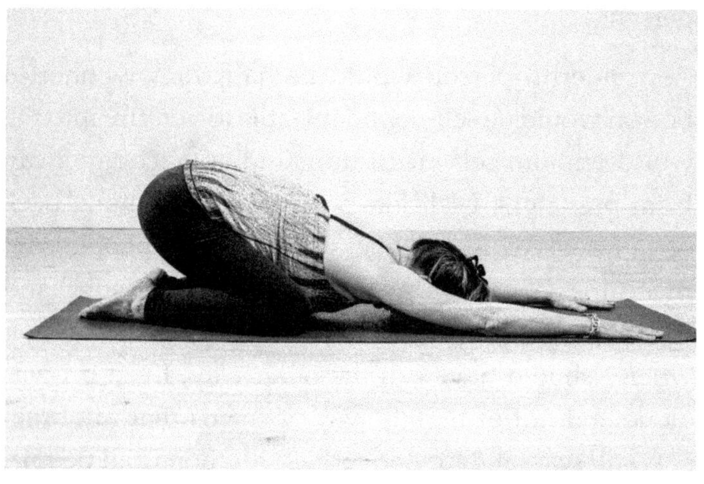

Yoga Pose: Child's pose helps to block out the external so we can go inward where it is safe and still.

Chapter 3:

Feeling Separate from Others

> *Ego Mantra: I am separate and alone.*
>
> *vs*
>
> *Heart Message: We are all connected.*

Yoga and Meditation Wisdom:

The Buddhist, Metta, prayer is very powerful in helping us to feel connected to others. Feeling that we are not separate. Feeling that the entire world is woven together and we are one of the threads.

Metta Prayer:

May we all be safe and protected;
May we all be pleased and content;
May our bodies be strong to support us;
And
May our lives evolve easily and effortlessly.

How will I ever fit in?

Marianne Williamson is one of my favourite authors and her books helped me to recover from my inner-critic and sort out why I really felt separate and alone. Williamson has written several books centered on the concepts found in *A Course in Miracles*. She is brilliant and much needed in today's world of "us vs them" mentality; binary thinking which unfortunately often ends in violence. I relate to almost everything found in the *Course* and Williamson's books, but I especially relate to the idea of feeling separate from others because I fear something about the interaction. Fear or love are the two main choices we have in life when we're reacting to people, places, and things. Past trauma made me, and countless others, react from a place of fear most of the time.

Feeling separate from others usually takes two forms: feeling either less than or more than someone else. I usually felt less than others. I could not relate to their world.

When you feel that you are less than others, your expectations for your life and what you can achieve are greatly affected. In the case of people who have witnessed conflict and experienced trauma, the world can be a dark place that is full of shame and isolation. The irony is that their very lack of connectedness can lead them to conclude that others don't experience pain in the same way. I thought that those around me, including my close friends, did not feel as much emotional pain as I did, that I was different. In reality, everyone suffers pain in his or her own way; our suffering is our shared humanity.

I hid my real feelings of being alone and exhausted. If I bought something new to wear, I would feel it wasn't as good as other people's clothing. If someone offered me some encouragement or a kind word, I would not trust them. Sometimes, I would give a compliment in the hopes of receiving one in return. I felt separate from the shiny, happy people. If I wasn't such a people-pleaser, I am sure I would have joined a counterculture group when I was in high school. I would have shunned social convention and approval, but I was hooked.

From the outside, I looked like I was fitting in. But, inside, I was afraid that I would be found out for the fraud that I thought I was. I would try new things at high school like joining a sports team or group but quit shortly after making the cut. I felt different and I gave up before I was found out. My internal judge and critic were always telling me that I would be discovered soon, so I should give up before that happened. It was no wonder that I gravitated toward alcohol. Having a few drinks allowed my inner world to be quiet for a while. I felt lighter when drinking with my girlfriends. Thank goodness for my beautiful friends, the bond between us is still strong today. If there was a ray of sunshine in my life at the time, it came from them.

When my first serious boyfriend came along, he gave me a form of validation that I very much needed. But I was unable to get close to him emotionally because he wanted a family and marriage. I was afraid that I couldn't measure up as a mother or wife. I wasn't worthy of a happy home with my husband and kids. I felt separate from the other women my age who were certain that they wanted to get married and have a family. I hid my true feelings of uncertainty behind feminism. I adopted the position that I wanted to wait to get married and have children until after I was established in a job. At the time, the economy was booming and a well-paying job wasn't hard to find. I would sabotage my enviable job in the end. I just couldn't believe that I could have the shiny, sparkly family and I feared that my job performance was not up to snuff either. If I am beginning to sound like I was Eeyore from Winnie the Pooh, that's because I *was.*

Later, my personal CBT and mindfulness practices taught me to start identifying what I thought about most of the time. Thoughts determine behaviour and action, they come from the core beliefs we have about life and ourselves. My thoughts were mostly negative and critical, so I believed I didn't deserve happiness. I would sabotage anything good that came into my life. I believed that I shouldn't stay at a job for any length of time because I would be exposed as a bad person. I am sure that my feelings of being bad stem from my past trauma; perhaps I thought that I had caused my family conflict.

I would change jobs, careers, every two years. I would sabotage relationships. I would allow myself to get only so close and then I would back off. I believed that distance in my relationships would protect me from harm. Being aloof and non-committal allowed me to leave the relationship at any time. Or, if I was exposed as not being nice, not being perfect, I could easily run away because my emotional investment was low. I only put any real effort into the relationships with my friends and then experienced tremendous loss when they got engaged to be married. The relationship would naturally change and I would miss the strong bond and connection we had.

The problem with feeling separate and afraid, is that it doesn't matter what you do or accomplish, you will never fully connect to a person, a group, or a job. I left my boyfriend and good job behind. I fooled myself into thinking I was leaving because there were better things to be discovered elsewhere, even though it meant being away from everything that meant anything to me: my hometown, my parents, my friends, and my boyfriend. I felt like Mary Richards from The Mary Tyler Moore show, the hit sitcom at the time.

I could act bubbly and be ambitious just like Mary was. Like her, I could leave my small town to make it on make own. On one hand, it felt wonderful to leave because I could finally be separate from everyone. On the other hand, I longed to feel less alone, more connected. I wanted to belong. Maybe it would happen in the new city I was moving to, or with the new friends I would make there. Just maybe, maybe, maybe. At least there was a sliver of hope that something could happen to make me feel less alone.

Today, I believe that glimmer of hope saved my life.

Yoga: Yoga helped me begin to relax enough so I could monitor my constant, fearful thoughts and question why I was having them when there was no danger around.

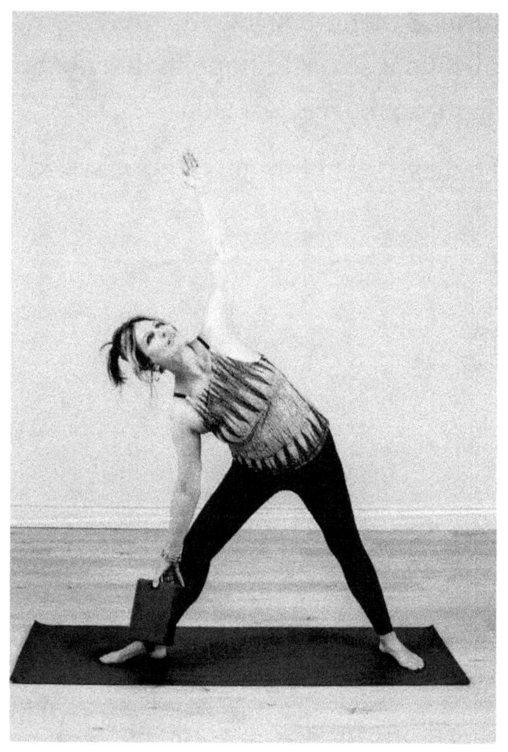

Yoga Pose: Triangle pose helps me to stretch and open my heart. With an open heart I notice when I am at my limit and cannot extend any further. I am gentle with my body.

Chapter 4:

Impression Management

Ego Mantra: No one will like the real you.

vs

Heart Mantra: We are all loveable and perfect!

Yoga and Meditation Wisdom:

Yoga, particularly Vipassana Yoga, which cultivates our non-judgmental inner witness, helps us to non-reactively become aware of everything that is happening in our life, of the thoughts we default to on a regular basis, and of how we are feeling inside. Mindful practices, which increase self-awareness, encourage us to cultivate the inner witness and to ACCEPT whatever we are thinking and feeling, rather than to run away from our feelings and thoughts. We learn that difficult emotions will dissipate after a short time if we allow them to surface. We can suffer, either for a longer period of time, by ignoring our feelings, or a shorter period, by acknowledging them. We have the choice.

I am not this hair, I am not this skin,
I am the soul that lives within.

Rumi.

How long can I keep fooling people?

I eventually came to realize that my prolonged effort of trying to manage people's impression of me, because I thought it would keep me safe, was, oddly enough, connected to my first Barbie doll. I also came to understand how all of my efforts to control others, which is another cognitive distortion, would lead me down the path to enlightenment.

I remember getting my first Barbie when I was about 6 years old. I wanted to be like Barbie. She looked perfect. She had the perfect figure, jobs, boyfriend, and bestie. Ken and Midge were her constant pals. Barbie could change how people viewed her simply by changing her outfits. If she wanted to be a cowgirl and have a horse, she could. If she wanted to be a nightclub singer, she could. I just changed her clothes. In real life, changing how people think of you is much more complicated. Still, I tried to convince others that I was nice and pleasant, and that I followed the rules.

I wore the clothes that they wore. I got the same haircut. I even wore the same amount of make-up as everyone else did. I tried to fit in and not make waves.

I continued to think that, if I dressed and talked like everyone else and had no problems, people would think that I was okay. I wasn't a freak and I wasn't loud or obnoxious in any way. I wanted to project that I was content and happy inside my skin. I wasn't one of those "angry feminists" that people made fun of at the time, though I held many of their views; views that had to be hidden. I only discussed socially acceptable topics that were light and non-confrontational. I guess that was why I was so drawn to the beer commercials of the time; everyone was easy going, having fun, and seemed to share a connection. I don't think that they have changed much. They still portray happy people, having a great time; the greatest time they have ever had in their life, in fact. I wanted to feel the same connection and camaraderie they were experiencing. Unfortunately, my experience was nothing like that. Of course, I had some wonderful, fun times with my girlfriends because we were all relaxed and safe. But, most of my drinking experiences were fraught with anxiety. I thought that my mask would slip and someone would notice that I wasn't quite as happy as I appeared to be while sober.

Despite my best efforts, my mask would slip at times and I became very sad and teary eyed. Where did this melancholia come from? I was just as surprised as everyone else was. I thought I was doing what I was supposed to be doing to be happy and content, however, I couldn't avoid feeling that I was grasping at straws. My life was no happy-go-lucky beer commercial. Still, instead of questioning the validity of their premise, I blamed myself for not living up to expectations. The only explanation I could come up with was that I was defective and needed to do more to control myself.

Still, some awareness was emerging. I became aware of conflicting thoughts for the first time and noticed my anger. I began to realize that I was suppressing my true feelings, thoughts, and actions. I was betraying myself and creating a very angry person in the process. This insight was very scary. Society fears female anger and it has found many ways to suppress and discourage it. I feared my anger, too.

The truth is that I wasn't doing a very good job of managing people's impressions of me. My anxiety, upset stomach, shortness of breath, and cold sores kept betraying me. They wouldn't go away. My body was trying to tell me something was wrong. It was trying to get my attention. It was trying to tell me that by not speaking my truth when I had the chance, I was not honouring my genuine, authentic Self.

The first clue that my efforts to control others' impressions weren't working for me came from a colleague. Someone I worked with at the time, compared me to a very strong woman on television. It seemed that I had successfully pulled off projecting the image of a confident female in control of her life, but the words rang hollow and I felt as plastic as Barbie on the inside. I felt terrible. As I sat with what he said and how it made me feel, I knew I was not being my true Self. Upon reflection, that was when I clearly heard the message that my soul had been trying to send me, for the first time. It was trying to help me see through my plastic façade and pay attention to the perfect luminous being each of us carries inside ourselves. Not Barbie or Ken perfect; something far better.

As my colleague's comment seeped through my denial and emotional armor, my anger started to bubble up. It terrified me at first, but I couldn't ignore it. After some real soul-searching I got honest with myself and decided to quit drinking. The floodgates opened. No longer held at bay by alcohol, sadness and grief welled up to the surface from the depths of my body. It was terrifying. Surprisingly, I knew I could handle whatever was coming up, the feelings would not engulf or paralyze me. I was going through a mid-life crisis of sorts. I couldn't push it away and I didn't want to. I knew I was entering a transformation process. My true Self was emerging.

I started to attend 12-step support group meetings and reading as many self-help books as I could get my hands on. I also began going to different body practitioners. Yoga reappeared in my life. I stopped attending business functions that served alcohol and fed my need for approval. I had to stand by the decision I had made to turn my life around. I had to stand in my truth.

I had disconnected from my drinking buddies. It was difficult. I was risking the disapproval of others. I often felt alone and unsure of myself, but I persevered. With each small step that I took toward finding out who I really was, I felt more cohesive, more whole. Little by little, I was stripping away old messages and expectations. I was finally on my soul's true path, which is not always easy, but always worth the journey.

Yoga: Paying attention to our body's comfort level and limitations during a yoga practice helps our authentic selves feel safe enough to emerge. We are listening to our body and heart when we only stretch or hold a pose to our edge and there is no pain. We clear a path for our luminosity to shine through.

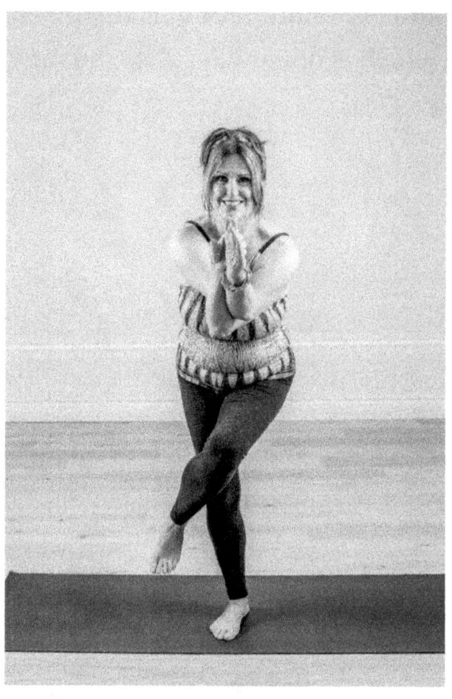

Yoga Pose: Eagle pose helps us to develop laser focus and vision. And, clarity.

Part 2:

Undoing Problematic Thinking: Going from "Not-my-day to Namaste"

There is a candle in your heart,
ready to be kindled.

There is a void in your soul, ready
to be filled.

You feel it, don't you?

Rumi.

What I did to begin feeling safe and more serene.

Hip, hip, hurrah, the healing and feeling better begins!

In this part of the book, I focus on the techniques that helped me to heal and some "Eureka" moments I had along the way. I talk about how I managed my anxiety through positive self-talk and finally stopped believing that what others think of me is more important than what I think of myself.

You will learn about the connection between anxiety and trauma and I will cover what worked for me and what I hope will be helpful for you too. If nothing else, I want to inspire you to really listen to your body and your intuition. I encourage you to go ahead and find solutions that suit you. Don't be afraid to adjust and tweak the techniques until they feel true and genuine for you. We are all unique and we are our own best therapist, guru and coach. I have found that wisdom will shine through if we are gentle with ourselves. Your next step will be revealed to you.

This is also the story of how yoga and mindfulness practices used in CBT and meditation come together in a wonderful healing mix. The body/mind connection is truly remarkable.

One of the key actions I took that helped me begin to see my light and feel more serene, was to return to regular yoga practice.

In addition to helping me stretch and become more flexible, breathe more deeply, and relax more, I found that it helped me to go beyond my physical body and connect with my inner world. Marion Woodman's books were instrumental in helping me to bridge the gap between my physical body and my inner domain. She honours the intuitive, feminine aspect of ourselves and describes how important it is to expect and listen for messages coming from within.

Getting in touch with our spirit is as important as connecting with the body. And do you know what the portal to our spirit is? Our body, of course! It therefore made sense that accepting and honouring my body would give me access to my interior world. The body is the gateway and the sensor of our exterior, which affects our interior landscapes. It needs to be acknowledged. Have you ever met someone and just had an uncomfortable or upset feeling in your stomach? That is your body reacting to your environment. What it is saying will depend on the circumstances but it is sending you a signal. Listen to it.

In Buddhism, there is the idea that somewhere in our body lies our luminous Self, which needs to be acknowledged and embraced, while the Ego is all about fear and likes to feel separate. This philosophy made sense to me on an emotional level; I found it very healing. I was attracted to the idea that my luminous Self wanted to express itself and was always waiting to be called upon. It gave me hope.

I also discovered that accepting my body was the first step in accepting my entire being, inside and out. Learning to be completely present during yoga helped to refresh my tired body and calm my worried mind. It also helped to reduce my fears about being imperfect. Yoga instructors asked me to go within to get in touch with whatever I was feeling and thinking. They also suggested that I accept whatever was presenting itself, then bid it farewell. It was like watching clouds passing by in my mind and not judging or resisting them.

I was finally allowing my light-filled, wonderful Self to peek through the clouds. In between breaths and in between thoughts, I was feeling calmer. My wonderful yoga teachers suggested I keep coming back to my breath and accept if it was difficult to do. It was like there was an umbrella of total acceptance above and within that was giving me permission to just be, just be myself.

I was giving myself permission to be with and accept whatever was coming up. I believe that my luminous Self was beginning to heal me from within. I have since learned that my luminous Self is always calm and steady, whereas my ego is full of chatter and worry. After only a short time of sitting quietly and being with my thoughts, a sense of peace would wash over me. My breathing became calmer. I was accepting whatever emotional or physical pain came up.

Physical pain is often easier to endure and acknowledge than emotional pain. My lower back, which had hurt for a long time, felt better after I finally admitted that it was tender. The stiffness and tenderness dissipated a bit after I accepted it was there and that I had past emotional baggage to address. Some people report radical healing after accepting their pain, but I held onto mine. According to self-help guru, Louise Hay, lower back problems have something to do with the past and lack of acceptance. I am sure there were many things I wasn't accepting and was in denial about at the time, but I was beginning to feel more hopeful about my future.

Forgiveness and acceptance are essential for healing past wounds; to this day, they are still central to my journey.

Yoga Wisdom: Our bodies and our minds are not our enemy. They are connected and need to be cared for.

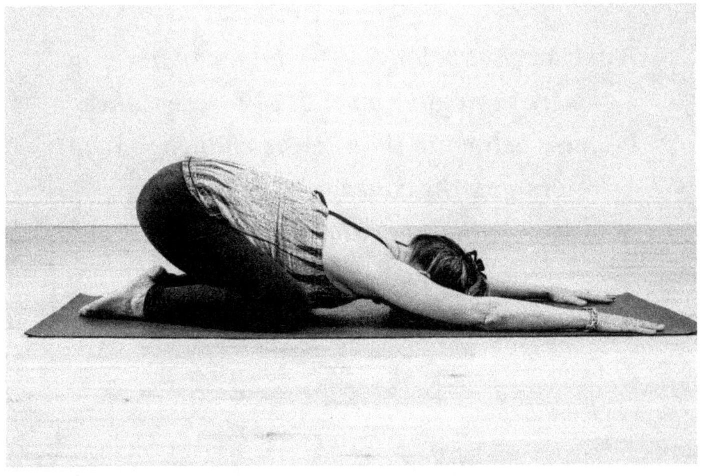

Yoga Pose: Remaining longer and more often in Child's Pose felt safe and allowed more thoughts and feelings to surface. I realized they were not that scary after all.

Chapter 5

Acceptance and Trust

> *The truth is: belonging starts with self-acceptance.*
> *Your level of belonging, in fact, can never be greater than your level of self-acceptance, because believing that you're enough is what gives you the courage to be authentic, vulnerable and imperfect.*
>
> **- Brene Brown -**

Yoga Wisdom:

Yoga and life are practices we do. We return to the mat as we show up for life: again, and again, and again. Maybe I don't accept myself every minute of every day, but I keep trying.

After giving up drinking, I still felt that I needed to do more to fully heal emotionally and physically. I had removed alcohol from my life to gain some much-needed clarity but it wasn't until much later that I realized *that all* of my self-destructive behaviors had been blocking my clarity and self-acceptance. The importance of self-acceptance crystallized for me one day when I came across a saying pasted to a washroom wall, of all places. It said:

Enough:

I am enough,

I do enough,

I have enough.

I tried to find out who had authored the quote but was not successful. Whatever its origin, I think it sums up how we should live our lives each moment of the day. How peaceful we would be if we were able to accept ourselves so unconditionally. We would accept and be satisfied with what we have in life, rather than strive to "keep up with the Jones." We would accept the intelligence, personality, and quirky traits that make us unique. Advertisers could no longer push products on us because we wouldn't worry about not being slim, pretty, handsome, or healthy enough.

That feeling of total self-acceptance is epitomized by the fictional character, Winnie-the-Pooh. Winnie-the-

Pooh seems to love and accept himself as he is. We don't hear Winnie complaining that he is too fat or has eaten too much honey. He seems to flow with whatever his life brings him. I wonder if Pooh has managed to learn some fundamental lessons that still elude us. I wonder if what life puts before us is for our greater good. Could our life journey be about learning to accept ourselves completely?

I came to understand that I was practicing radical self-acceptance during one of the most stressful periods of my life. It happened when I went through the process of selling and buying a house. That was when I realized that fear can be triggered whenever our security is threatened. What could be more basic to our security than shelter?

I had convinced my husband that buying and selling our homes was a good way to save up enough money for me to take early retirement from my government job, and that's what we did. So far our efforts had been successful; our homes had sold fast and the ones we purchased had all been good investments. On this occasion, we decided that we would sell our current home and downsize once again. We would bank most of the funds and add to our nest egg.

The market was very hot but the problem came when we decided to sell at a slow time of the year for family homes like ours. Families had already moved so their children could start school in September. Our home was very desirable and should have sold in record time; however, with September just around the corner, it sat for a while. We had planned a short vacation in mid-September, thinking that it would have sold by then. It hadn't.

We went on our 10-day holiday, filled with anxiety and uncertainty. Having read many self-help books, I believed that lessons came in many forms, which gave me hope. I knew there was a lesson to be gained from the delay in selling our beautiful home, my favourite so far. To soothe my anxiety, I would go sit in nature.

I had also begun to do daily affirmations and positive self-talk. I kept up a constant mantra: "I let go and trust the universe will provide me with whatever is for the greatest good." I was prepared to keep our home and flip the other one we had purchased, if need be. Although that would not have been the ideal outcome.

I felt badly because my husband trusted my decision-making ability when it came to buying and selling houses. I experienced tremendous anxiety thinking about how I had let him down. I was still a people-pleaser at heart and it was emotionally painful for me to think that I had thrown a wrench into our plans. I tried not to doubt my/our decision to sell our beautiful home but nevertheless felt great insecurity around it. My inner critic began to take over.

While we were on our holiday, something terrible happened. I chipped my tooth on a plastic fork, which caused me enormous physical pain. My root was exposed and it made me cringe at the slightest bit of pressure or airflow. Louise Hay says that tooth issues are linked to indecision or feeling that you have made the wrong decision. Wow, that was exactly how I felt. I was trying to eat breakfast one day after it happened and I started to cry in the restaurant. Ian was shocked because I rarely cried. I was taking on all the responsibility for making what seemed to be a very bad decision to sell the house and feeling terrible about it.

He had also agreed to the sale, but I felt that it was primarily my fault. To counteract the pain I was in, both emotionally and physically, I doubled-down on my mantra, saying it over and over again. I trusted that the situation was playing out exactly as it should so I could learn a valuable life lesson. I began to feel a little better after he agreed to cut our 10-day trip to 7 days. We were able to book an early flight home without financial penalty, which also helped my outlook. I got the tooth looked at when we got home but could not get it extracted for another few days. I felt vulnerable and very critical of myself. I was emotionally and physically beaten up; not exactly a model for self-acceptance and trust. All the while, my spouse wasn't blaming me for anything. I was terrorizing myself, a familiar feeling.

Finally, we got an offer on the house and we accepted it. Thankfully, by that time, I had accepted that I had done nothing wrong in wanting to put the house up for sale and that my intentions had been good. In the end, everything turned out for the better. The decision to sell, allowed us to build a home two years down the road. The equity we gained from downsizing, allowed us to use our nest egg for the building process.

Although I was shaky at times, I managed to hold on to my belief that the Universe had a better plan for me than I could ever have imagined, and it came true. Valuable lessons were learned, not the least of which was that trust and acceptance work hand-in-hand. I learned to trust the decision I had made, accept whatever was happening in the moment, and to stand firm on future decisions. As long as I make them with careful and deliberate thought, without intentionally hurting anyone, I can relax and trust myself.

Fast forward to the future for a lesson in vulnerability. Author Brené Brown writes about how vulnerability threatens our sense of safety and security. I have certainly found this to be true in my life. I learned all about vulnerability and my ability to sit with the feeling on the day I went to my post-graduate interview. The interview would determine whether I was suitable enough, smart enough, *something* enough, to enter my first post-graduate program. My vulnerability and insecurity came in part from my status as a mature student. I had learned the hard way that being older than the majority of other students didn't guarantee that I would do better.

My husband dropped me off. I remember being very nervous yet calm at the same time. As we pulled up my heart began beating faster and louder. I turned to him and said, "You know this is about something bigger and more important than if I get into graduate school." He replied, "Yes." Ian is very astute. For me, it was about being vulnerable, not in full control, and feeling the full extent of my insecurities, but going forward anyway. It was about knowing that other people had control over me. It was scary, but I had decided to *trust*. I didn't have a back-up plan if I didn't get in. Regardless of the outcome, I trusted that I was going to be okay. I realized that even if I wasn't accepted into the program, I was proud of the progress I had made in school. I could write better, engage in critical thinking, and make presentations to an audience.

As I walked down the hall to the interview, I remembered another time when I had felt total shame and embarrassment at school; it was after finding out that I had received a low grade. I was attending community college on a part-time basis while I worked full-time. I had to take an Economics class for my business certificate and I barely passed. I received the test back and went to the washroom, where I put my head in my hands and started to cry. I was so ashamed. At the time, I had no positive self-talk to help alleviate the disappointment I felt. For me, the poor grade just confirmed how little I knew and that I shouldn't have taken the program. I was devastated. I felt that I wasn't as smart as I had thought. It took me a long time to get over that mark and be vulnerable enough to go talk to the teacher about how I could improve. To my credit, I continued with the class and eventually passed the program with honours. We all excel at different things; economics was not my best subject.

Today, the memory of that event makes me so thankful that I have improved my self-talk. Now, I try to catch myself when I am feeling insecure. I take care of the wounded part of me that has been triggered. In the past, I would have continued my negative thoughts and spiralled down in shame and I would have engaged in some, unhealthy, distracting behaviour. Also, even if I was unaware of it at the time, that experience was an exercise in vulnerability, to the extent that I went and got the help I needed from my teacher despite how I felt. I was able to be vulnerable and still come out the other side stronger than I had been going in.

The memory of that past event, and my eventual triumph over shame, gave me strength as I headed into the interview. This time, I would go in with eyes wide open to my vulnerability and use it to help me be my authentic Self. I sat in front of a panel of professors and spoke my truth, which included informing them that I was nervous; something I would not have been able to do without practising self-acceptance and trusting that everything would work out. I was accepted into the post-graduate program.

My critical self-talk was being replaced with more loving, heart-centered thoughts, which was having a positive effect on my life and creating better outcomes. It was a process that happened over time, after I prioritized monitoring my self-talk. It also became easier for me to accept my vulnerability because, having quieted my inner-critic and negative thoughts, I could now imagine positive results.

While writing this chapter at a local coffee shop, I spilled a plastic container of trail mix that I carry with me for instant energy. Instead of getting upset and down on myself, I scooped up the spill and put it in the garbage. No negative self-talk was heard. I like to celebrate these little victories when they happen.

Fast Track Your Healing - Acceptance:

If there is something I could wrap around me or cozy up with, it is acceptance.

Acceptance helps us stay in the moment and flow with whatever is happening in our life at any given time.

Change is the only constant, which is why acceptance is so important. If I resist what is happening or what someone is saying to me, I am going against the reality of the moment. Taoist thought is all about flowing in, and with, the stream of life. Its ebb and flow, its ups and downs.

Falling short when our best efforts fail can put a dent in our emotional well-being —acceptance and trusting it will all work-out in the end, helps to build resiliency after disappointment.

Yoga: I accept that on some days I do a strong, flowing series of Sun Salutations. And that, on other days, not so much. A mantra which helps this process, "I accept me."

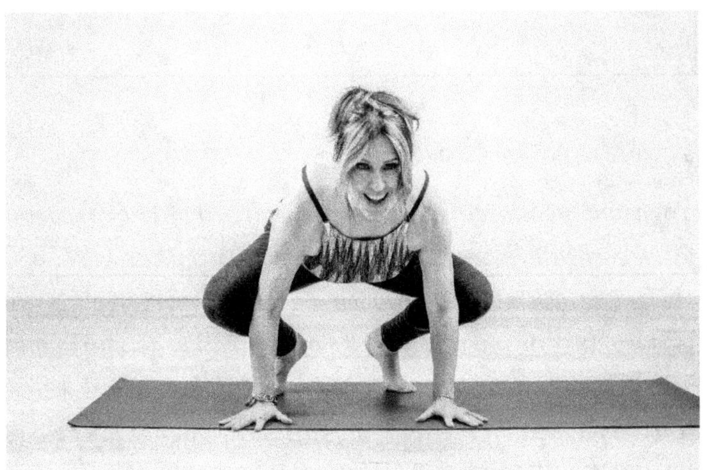

Yoga Pose: I keep trying to do Crow Pose which is a difficult pose for me and accept whatever the outcome. I am afraid of tipping over and falling face forward to the ground, but I still give it a try when it comes up in class.

Chapter 6:
Self-Criticism and Judgment

> *Until you make the unconscious conscious,*
> *it will direct your life and you will call it fate.*
>
> *- Carl Jung –*

Yoga/Meditation Wisdom

Yoga and meditation helped me to realize that I have several fear-based, negative, and critical voices within me. So, I started to ask questions when I was not happy with my performance or my reaction. I would breathe, get quiet, and ask if my response had been appropriate. Was I being reasonable and loving with myself? Who among my cast of inner characters was doing the talking? Could I be more kind to myself? More accepting? Or, did I need to apologize for my actions and not feel ashamed for having to do so?

Bringing our seemingly disparate selves together—Forgiveness of Self comes first!

Buddhist meditation asks us to cultivate a non-judgmental inner witness. It suggests that we become aware of our normal "go-to" thoughts and feelings. CBT also suggests we monitor our thoughts, feelings, and our subsequent actions. This is all very time consuming and quite tedious at times. I wanted a quick fix but I found that it wasn't that easy. Whenever I took any notice of my thoughts I found a massively dominant inner critic and stern judge lurking in the background. There was also a very prissy, uptight prude who was constantly on guard, watching to see if I behaved properly, like a "lady" would.

And, what was the common denominator behind all that judgment and criticism? Fear.

After trying different personal growth exercises and steps, I found that my ability to remain non-judgmental and less fearful increased when I began reading Debbie Ford's work. Ford focused on the inner energies that rule our life based on past conditioning and messages received during childhood. Her ideas shared similarities with Carl Jung's group of sub-personalities. I came across another, similar, concept in Family Systems psychotherapy and the work of Hal and Didra Stone, in the form of internal personalities vying for dominance. A deeper process started within me when I identified the different selves that were running my show. Based on the advice of the authors, I worked to make friends with my inner selves and glean from them whatever wisdom I could. Apparently, my cast of characters needed to be heard and listened to. Change did not happen overnight, but, over time, I began to see some progress. As the frustrating 12-Step saying goes, "it takes as long as it takes" to start to heal.

The first personality I came across was the very bossy "inner critic." Nothing was right for this little perfectionist. She was driving the bus and the others were trying to be heard, but she was having no part of it. Even the parts of me that were kind and caring were drowned out by this loudmouth.

It was very hard for me to embrace this side of myself. She was loud, obnoxious, and very, very controlling. She would lord it over the others and have them march to her tune. After several attempts, I finally got her to let down her guard. She appreciated that she was no longer being drowned out with alcohol, shopping, or being busy most of the time, but, she would only agree to talk to me if I allowed her to control the flow of conversation. I did.

During a visualization exercise where my entire cast of characters were present, she finally answered my questions. After more reassurance and understanding, we finally had a free flowing and fruitful conversation. I asked her to explain a few things: why are you here in this important position? In a position that rules me? Why do you need to be so vigilant in your efforts to stay in control? The answers came fast and furious, but the gist was that she wanted to stay in control at all times because if she did not, we would be hurt, embarrassed, or fail. She was convinced that I would be tromped on by people, jobs, or situations.

My inner critic felt that my other "selves" were too weak and trusting. She knew how to take care of me, especially "Little Holly." Little Holly was wounded. She was frightened of everyone and everything. She needed protecting. My inner critic would also protect me from the other parts of myself that did not feel good enough or deserving of happiness or success. She was helping me not to be exposed. I had to hand it to her, she had my back and she popped up whenever a new person or position was presented to me. After a few more visualization exercises, I understood and trusted that she was Little Holly's protector. I once had a dream that a little girl had just been raped and was lying in a heap of rubble. I saw her through a window and wanted to go and get her but decided not to. Now I felt that I should embrace her and that if I did, perhaps my inner critic would lessen her grip on me.

I began by trying to have a conversation with Little Holly and offered to come and get her away from the stones and the broken building she was in. I am sure that I was the broken building. After some time, she agreed to let me in and offered me her hand. This was an important and powerful moment in my recovery. I knew that I was on the right track when my inner critic allowed me to take her hand. I brushed off the rubble and gave her a big hug. She was shivering. I instantly loved her and she seemed to connect with me. I somehow knew that she was part of the luminous being within that I was born to reclaim and love. She was bruised and scraped. I helped her up and we went outside. The sun hurt her little eyes, but she was glad she was helped out from under the broken bricks.

I believe we all have scared little boys and little girls within us, waiting to be acknowledged and cared for.

I can't say that I never abandoned her again, but at least I was aware that she was within me and needed to be noticed and loved in a kind and tender way. Love for my wounded inner child came by way of rest, nutrition, compassion, and going back to school. After some time I acknowledged that I was capable and enjoyed learning. I realized I could go back to school and get something that I always wanted to get, a university degree. This would validate Little Holly and allow her to be more authentic, be her true self. She was bright and loved to help people but could only do so if she stopped criticizing herself and took some chances. A university degree would put her in a better position to help others.

Once I got in touch with my inner child, my inner critic relaxed, and so did my inner perfectionist. I was able to make some mistakes and not beat myself up over them. My need to control people, places and things eased up as well. I didn't need to control my environment so tightly to feel safe. At times, when my anxiety was at its height, I would envision wrapping Little Holly in my arms and gently rocking her. I felt immediate release from the tension and turmoil I was experiencing. I can still feel instant fear and panic, but these episodes are decreasing in intensity and duration as I continue to nurture myself with loving thoughts.

In addition to having tools to stop or decrease the intensity of my panic attacks, I began feeling that it was okay to take more risks. As with the negative domino effect that I had experienced in the past, one thing led to another, but this time it was a *positive* domino effect. I wasn't perfect, nor was anyone else for that matter. I was human. I had good and bad days. I realized I had anger, sadness, even joy, within. I was trying to accept all of my feelings and by doing so keep my inner critic and anxiety at bay. She didn't have to protect me against feeling stupid or embarrassed because I had accepted that we all make mistakes. Mistakes meant that I was human and just like everyone else on the planet. I felt a part of the human race for the first time. I was connected and not separate. I was not alone.

I worked to uncover all of the hidden parts of myself. After a while, the cast of characters I discovered were actually *fun*. They all had a good sense of humour, including my inner critic who was the queen and boss lady. I noticed more small changes. It felt okay to meet new people and not hurry away for fear of exposure. I was also less rigid when shopping for new clothes. I didn't have to have the perfect colour dress to match my purse and shoes. I was relaxing and becoming the Self that I always wanted to be. A more peaceful, accepting Self. According to Buddhist thought, I have always been kind and loving but had to discover that part of my Self where real perfection and acceptance lies.

Fast Track Your Healing: WTF or Why the Forgiveness?

Forgiving your Self opens up healing and frees you from the damage created by your inner critic and judge.

Holding grudges and resentments against others and ourselves is not only draining but also a waste of time. It keeps us separate from others, fearful and very defensive.

Moreover, holding on to resentment produces extremely negative energy and releases the stress hormone, Cortisol. It is toxic for our body. In other words, the most important "F" word is Forgiveness.

One of the most powerful 12-step program sayings I have ever heard is "Allowing someone to live in your head rent free is only harming YOU!" Words to live by.

You forgive for your own peace of mind, not anyone else's. Until you can forgive yourself, or someone else, you are not free to live your life. By doing so, you are not condoning bad behaviour you are freeing yourself and are no longer a prisoner of your negative feelings. Forgiveness and acceptance go hand in hand. When you forgive you are accepting what has happened and choosing to view your situation from a new perspective. You become less negative and it softens you.

Yoga: When I wear mismatched socks, no make-up, or take a rest during class I know I am accepting myself completely. The perfectionist and inner critic are no longer driving the bus. They are still inside me but accept they don't need to take control.

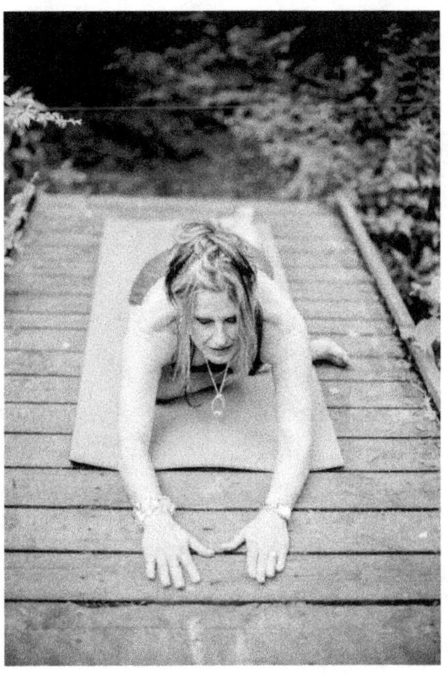

Yoga Pose: Pigeon Pose is hard on my knees and when they are hurting I need to let up and switch my mind-set from trying to be perfect to being kind to myself. Self-compassion is all important.

Chapter 7

Not Over-Personalizing

> **Let silence take you to the core of life.**
>
> **- Rumi -**

Yoga Wisdom:

The only thing you can control is your present thought. Choose wisely.

Feeling More at Peace

Giving up alcohol and doing yoga again on a regular basis was a huge boost to my healing but there was still a lot of work for me to do. I needed to go deeper. I was still hyper-vigilant and overly worried about how I was coming across to people and how they were reacting to me. I was easily hurt by what others said and still believed that they were trying to upset me. After I became a therapist and began working with clients who had also experienced trauma I explored trauma and its effects more fully. Eventually, I realized that I was really doing the research for me. I needed to learn more for my own mental health.

Feeling safe is important when it comes to living with the effects of past trauma. I already recognized on a superficial level that over-personalizing, or taking things too personally, was connected to my need to keep safe by controlling the environment around me. Distraction is also an important coping mechanism and focusing on others and what they were thinking was a way for me to keep my mind *very* busy and avoid my past trauma.

When I began to dig into the subject of trauma during my post-graduate studies, I was very drawn to vicarious trauma and did a paper on it. I was working in the family violence field at the time and wondered if volunteers experienced trauma through hearing and reading the stories of victims of domestic abuse. I was volunteering at a men's domestic violence agency and thought that I was immune to vicarious trauma because I had done some inner child work—thank-you John Bradshaw – and had already acknowledged the domestic violence I had witnessed in my home. Back then, I thought the main take-away from these frightening experiences was that I had potential trust issues when it came to people who I thought had control over me, such as bosses and my spouse. My parents had been distracted and embroiled in their conflict, which left me feeling abandoned at times and unsafe in the relationship.

Later, I realized that the trauma I had experienced had affected me far more than I originally thought and that my preoccupation with the opinion of others was one of its consequences. I was always worrying about what others were thinking of me because I needed them to like me. Through my research I learned that, in my mind, if they liked me, I would feel safe. My sympathetic nervous system would not be triggered because there would be no threat of danger, which meant that it would not spring to action to heighten my senses, increase my heartbeat, and make my breathing shallow to conserve my energy. The mind is a powerful thing.

I was always on guard for the slightest hint of rejection, disappointment, or disagreement. If I detected any, I would quickly try to remedy the situation as my anxiety started to escalate. I was better able to control my fear on some days than on others. It depended on the situation. I remember getting regular panic attacks when I entered the sales world. I would stress about not making enough sales calls that day, and so I would book too many calls. Then, I would be afraid that I wouldn't get to all of them in one day. And then, I would worry that if I *didn't* make them all, I was going to fail at my job and risk my bosses' disapproval, disappointment, and anger. I believed that if I disappointed someone it was a threat to my safety and as frightening as not being liked because I could not control how they would treat me.

I was anxious every single day I held that position, which was for years. Looking back, I believe that I was drawn to high-stress jobs because it kept that feeling of panic in my life. Being unable to control my environment at all times wasn't pleasant but stress was a familiar feeling. Safety and at ease were not. Since no one can possibly control their environment at all times, my brain interpreted many situations as assaults on my well-being and sense of security.

I had witnessed people in my home not being safe, myself included, and I carried that feeling out into the world each day. I have come to understand that feeling threatened and scared was imprinted on my brain. Typically, people who have experienced or witnessed traumatic events walk on eggshells most of the time, constantly worried. I would later learn an extremely valuable lesson: the only thing I *can* control is my reaction to what is happening.

My paper on vicarious trauma taught me to take care of myself and be mindful of whether or not I was over-reacting to situations at my family violence job. Given my background, over reacting could include sudden feelings of anger, sadness, or fear. I did not relate my panic and terror to trauma until much later.

Once I became a social worker, I wanted to bring awareness of PTSD to first responders and high stress workers. I wanted to help teach people about its symptoms and possible remedies. Little did I know that I was educating myself. I still thought that if I was aware of the potential to develop vicarious trauma and PTSD symptoms, I took care of myself, and was mindful going forward, I would not be affected. Meanwhile, I had been showing signs of trauma the entire time I was working in the family violence, addiction, and justice fields. I didn't feel safe. I had problems getting close to and trusting people. I finally realized that I had all of the symptoms of PTSD: I suffered from anxiety, intrusive thoughts, constant worry, physical pain, and an inability to concentrate, just to name a few.

My anxiety symptoms could not be ignored any longer. One day, I was driving to a post-graduate class and was overcome with full-blown panic and anxiety. I didn't want to go to class. I knew a group class assignment was coming up and I didn't want to do it. I could control my own work and submit it, but I was engulfed in fear at the thought of having to talk to and work with my classmates. I was afraid that they did not like me and thought I couldn't contribute much to the assignment.

My prehistoric brain went into full protection mode, making my breathing shallow and my senses hyper aroused. I felt that no one would want me in their group and, even if they did, they would not think I was smart enough. A familiar feeling surfaced, I felt like a huge fraud. I could not get my breathing back to normal. I gasped for air as I drove closer to the school parking lot. According to Linda Graham, an expert on resiliency, personal growth, and transformation, the brain searches for any possible type of threat to one's well being. That's what was happening to me at that moment but I didn't fully grasp what was going on. I later came to understand this process on a profoundly healing level.

Despite these very telling episodes, I still did not realize that I was suffering from symptoms of trauma. My fear response was confusing to me, and no doubt to others, because there was no direct threat to my physical well-being. The threat was to my emotional well-being and that's what was causing the stress. Thankfully we are learning more and more about trauma and its impact. I now believe that I suffered trauma in childhood because of the violence I witnessed in my home. That initial trauma was exacerbated over the years when I experienced fear from perceived threats in different social contexts. Trauma is cumulative and I have little doubt that a combination of minor physical and emotional threats, along with some major ones, continued to build the trauma over time. An ectopic pregnancy and subsequent close brush with death were definitely major attacks on my safety and it seems that my post-graduate group work was as well. I felt threatened at the thought of working closely with others and I panicked. I tried to give myself calming self-talk, but I was missing the key message I needed to deliver to my mind. I needed to say, "I am safe, I am safe." And, equally important, "I am not alone." But I didn't.

Thankfully, I had a tape in my car by Pema Chodron, a Buddhist nun who talks about the Bodhisattva, having compassion for others and yourself, and how we are all suffering in some way. She says that compassion and understanding are important to feeling better. It was playing but turned down low; I turned it up hoping it would distract me from my fear and panic. What I heard was that it is more important to give compassion to yourself before giving it to others. This is because, like love, you can't fully give it to another until and unless you have given it to yourself.

I am sure that I had heard these words before, but this time around they truly resonated with me. I began to breathe more deeply after listening to a few lines.

Realizing that many people around the world share the same emotions that I am having at any given moment, was a huge "a-ha!" moment for me. If true, I wasn't alone. There were others who felt separate and inadequate, who felt full-on fear and dread, who were having panic attacks. I self-reflected and understood why so many people self-soothe with alcohol, drugs, or any manner of distraction. I used to drink and I used to shop to feel better but neither of these coping mechanisms were truly effective. I was still afraid. Sometimes I even felt terror after a night of drinking because I worried about what I had said, how I had come across to others. Did I piss anyone off and would they hurt me somehow? I remember often having intense stomach cramps until I quit drinking completely. As I thought about how many people were going through the same thing as I was, I suddenly felt compassion for all of the times this had happened to me and to countless others.

As I drove and listened to the Chodron tape, I felt that we were all suffering together. In that moment of feeling connected to others I began accepting myself a little more and it felt good. I felt some peace sweep over me. I was not alone. I thought that there must be others in my post-grad program who were feeling the same way I did. It was a tough course that demanded huge amounts of time and attention. Other students in the program had very young families. It was difficult for all of us and I felt connected; we were all in this together. It was wasn't about me, it was about us.

After calming down by concentrating on my breath, I tried once again to give myself positive self-talk and reminded myself that each of us excels in some areas and not in others. It occurred to me that our group could work together to bring out the best qualities in each of us, in order to ensure that our assignment was a good one. I knew that education was really about self-growth and becoming a happier, healthier person. I knew that, if I pushed through, that would be the result. I still had a lot to work on, but I was feeling better and that gave me hope. I soothed my fear and panic by recognizing that there were other people who felt the same way I did. We understood each other. Feeling that connection diminished my anxiety, while my calm breath helped to produce quieter, more positive thoughts. I wasn't over-personalizing the group work any longer; I felt that we were a team.

Fast Track Your Healing

Thinking both my thoughts *and yours* is exhausting, so I endeavor to stop myself now.

Here is what I recommend if you want to fast track your healing in this area. First, try to be mindful about how you are reacting in any given situation. That way, if you need to, you can give yourself positive, loving affirmations that make you feel safe instead of growing anxious. The idea is to nip your fear in the bud before it escalates. If you don't catch it in time and some escalation occurs, remember that you are not alone, many others are feeling exactly the same way at that same moment.

Replace "I" thinking with "we."

Yoga: Some believe the longest distance to travel is from the head to the heart. Opening the front of our bodies helps to shorten the distance.

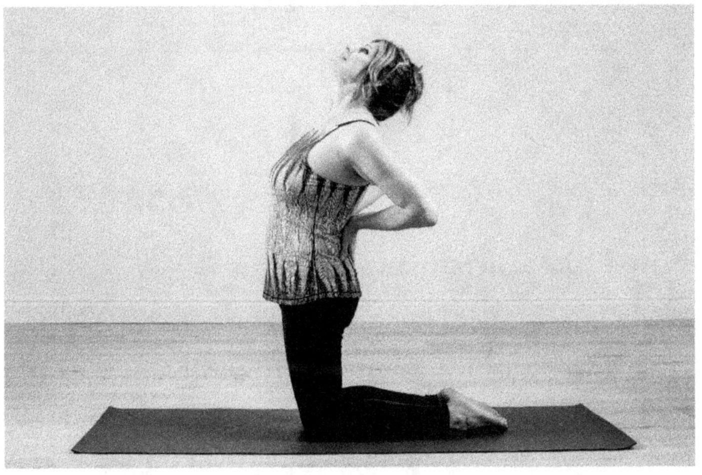

Yoga Pose: Doing back bends like Bow Pose helps me to open my heart and think more lovingly and less fearfully about myself and others.

Chapter 8:
Spirituality

Yoga Wisdom:

Yoga helps to bring together and unite body and spirit.

Why I like Christmas so much

I think this is a good time to mention spirituality and I don't necessarily mean religion. Spirituality was and continues to be an important part of my healing. In fact, a belief in something greater than myself that is helping me to navigate through life, has become the most important factor contributing to my feelings of safety and self-acceptance. Carl Jung wrote about meaningful coincidences and the fact that I am writing this chapter on December 24th holds much meaning for me. I love Christmas and always have. If we could relax our need to control every minute of our life to a higher power, we could achieve peace on Earth.

To me, Christmas is not about the material trappings and commercialism, it is about kindness and generosity. People are kinder and more generous during the holiday season and I have come to believe that this reflects our true spiritual nature. I also like to think that all of the beautiful Christmas lights displayed at that time of year are directing us toward the light that is within us. We are luminous beings. When ending a yoga class I always say, "Namaste," and the meaning of this word that I gravitate toward is, "The light within me, sees and blesses the light within each of you." When we look at the lights on a Christmas tree we catch a glimpse of the light within ourselves and our potential to love and forgive.

When I was young, my favourite Christmas decoration was a candle encircled by a ring of metallic angels. The heat generated by the candle made the angels spin. I would watch it for what seemed like hours. I was drawn to it because somehow I knew that we are more than our physical bodies. Angels are from the spiritual realm; I wonder if we are too? Many believe that we have angels watching over us all of the time and that we can call upon them to help us. They want to help us. I am sure that I unconsciously called on them many times in my life, especially when I had my close brushes with death.

So, if we are light-filled beings, what are we doing here on Earth? Why not be spiritual beings of light all of the time in another realm? I think it is because it takes time to fully realize our spiritual nature . We must first learn the lessons that life has to teach us. For me, this explains why there is so much suffering in the world, why there is abuse and poverty. The challenges we go through and the lessons we learn help us to become our most loving, light filled selves. People like Nelson Mandela and Ghandi were very advanced when it came to love and forgiveness. So was philosopher, Viktor Frankl. Frankl made a conscious decision to forgive his Nazi captors and treat them with respect and kindness. Suddenly, they treated him more humanely. They couldn't treat him in a subhuman manner any longer; he was a human being just like they were. These three examples are good role models for us to emulate as we strive to become more like our highest Self, our spirit.

I believe that I have only had one spiritual experience in my life. I was 22 years old and living in an apartment. I had just finished doing the laundry and I was alone, having a drink by my balcony door and looking at the night sky. Jon Anderson of the band, *Yes*, was playing in the background; his beautiful voice and lyrics transporting me to another realm. I felt peaceful as I turned in for the night. Some time later, I woke up to feeling myself being lifted toward the ceiling. From my elevated position, I could see the bed below. There were white daisies all around the edge of my bed. I felt as though I could transport myself anywhere. I believe that I was experiencing what is called astro-projection. I remembered having read about it and that it occurs most often during sleep. I suddenly got scared, and with a thud I was back in my body. There was tingling and bright lights for a few seconds after I returned. This was my only experience with astro-projection. I don't know if I shut it down or if it was only meant to be a one-time event.

For me, the effects of meditation on my life are evidence that I am, at least in part, spirit. I can meditate for 10 minutes in the morning and feel totally uplifted. I feel light and airy. I meditate on my luminous Self and on having perfect, optimal health. And, in fact, I rarely ever get sick, which I believe is linked to my daily mantra and prayer practice. I visualize being nurtured by Mother Earth. This nurturing fills my entire body with health and wellness. My bones, blood, veins, muscles, and skin are all nourished with love and health.

I truly believe that the time I spend in quiet prayer and meditation is enough to help me align with my spirit, my luminous Self. I feel safe. Knowing there is a higher power guiding my life helps me to get in touch with this beautiful, light-filled being that I am—that we all are. Some people liken the process to the peeling of an onion. We peel the layers back one by one until we finally get to the good stuff. We peel off our past conditioning and the messages that do not serve us well, until we finally reach our beautiful inner core. All of the negative and unloving self-talk is stripped away and replaced with positive thoughts and new core beliefs. That is when we start to believe and trust that we are innocent, loving, forgiving, pure beings.

My morning practice changes every few months but I usually start by giving thanks for the day ahead before

I even get out of bed. I then stretch for 10 minutes and spend 10 more minutes sitting quietly. I give more thanks for the blessings in my life and offer my service to help others. I pledge to be kind and forgive those that may annoy me during the course of the day. Some days are better than others. I offer to be a conduit for the Universe, so that God and the angels can work through me. Then, I might ask for something that I need; in the past, I have asked for more clients so that I can help more people. Or, I might ask for patience with someone I am having a problem with. I have also asked for material things, such as a new vehicle or a beautiful house near water and green space. Those requests were granted. In fact, almost everything I ask for manifests in some way.

My wellness ritual also includes walking outdoors a few times per week and being mindful. My mind still races sometimes, so I quiet my thoughts by focusing on my breath, my steps, or the colours I see around me. I breathe in the fresh air and I thank the Universe quite often during these walks.

The physical practices I engage in to keep me close to my spirit are yoga and the workouts I do with a fitness circle or stretch band a few times per week. I try to not race through my routine but often do; I am human and accept my restless mind. I have never been interested in taking a spin or boot camp class. Someone yelling at me is too scary and triggering for me. In order to help with my mental health and well-being, I try to reframe anything unpleasant that is happening so that I am better able to accept it. I try to see the lesson in it. I try to forgive any person I believe has offended me in some way. I also try to establish what part I played in creating the unpleasant situation, and how I can go forward as calmly as possible to achieve a positive outcome with the person involved. It isn't always easy but I keep trying and practicing.

I feel that my simple spiritual practice is yielding results; I am feeling more peace on Earth. I am more calm and accepting of myself. I am also getting bolder as I feel safe enough to venture out and take small risks. I am feeling more comfortable when talking to people and really connecting with them on a meaningful level. My daily ritual is pretty simple and, whatever else I do, I always take a moment to list who and what I am grateful for. I include my author mentors on that list: Louise Hay,

Marion Woodman, Marianne Williamson, Robert Holden, and Wayne Dyer, to name a few. My own practices are composites of what I have learned from them, over the years. These authors are remarkable angels. Sadly, some have departed but their work lives on through their writings.

Fast Track Your Healing

Spirituality is different for everyone.

It is important to find what works for you!

Spirit is always loving and kind. I know I am in contact with mine when I feel peaceful and calm.

Answers to questions come to me in a quiet way.

Our ego is always trying to control situations and shouting for us to try. We must surrender control and trust.

Yoga: Total relaxation of the body allows our higher power to heal us. All the stretching, strengthening, opening, and repairing are accelerated when we surrender.

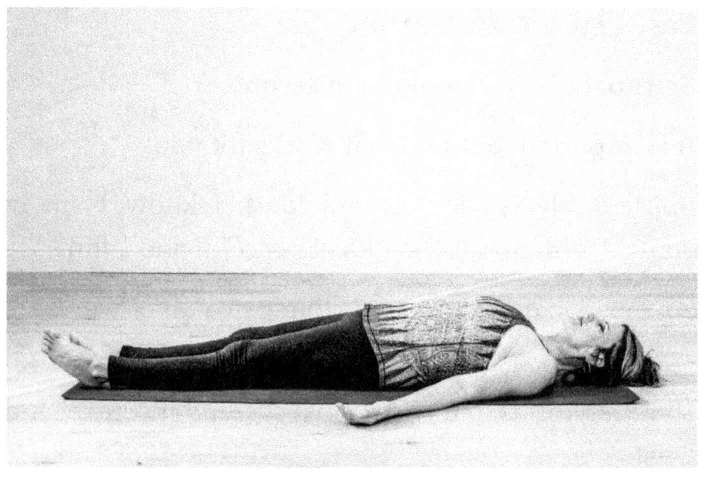

Yoga Pose: Shavasana or relaxation pose helps me to feel light and close to my Spirit.

Chapter 9:

Getting Quiet, Reframing, and Connecting

> *Your visions will become clear only when*
> *you can look into your own heart.*
> *Who looks outside, dreams;*
> *who looks inside, awakes.*
>
> *- Carl Jung –*

Yoga Wisdom:

Connection with Self happens in a group or in solitude, but we can't truly connect with others until we connect with our Self. Get quiet and still to feel the connection.

Getting quiet, reframing, and connecting to stay calm and deepen my spiritual Self

I have found that being still and quiet in our very busy and noisy world is powerful and spiritually uplifting. I searched for peace and connection to Self for years because I was so anxious as a child. I remember that I would often go for walks outside and deeply breathe in the air. It helped to quiet my mind. I would also soothe my soul with soft music.

Taking time to get quiet and still is very important for our mental health and well-being, a lesson I learned early on. In my 20s I was working two waitressing jobs to pay my rent. I was working a split shift, waiting on tables during the busy lunch hour into the afternoon at one restaurant, then going home for a break before starting the night shift at another. I would leave my first job around 4pm and arrive home already exhausted, knowing that I had to go out again. But, after lying on the couch, putting my feet up on the back, resting my eyes, and getting quiet, I would feel reenergized. I could always rely on this technique of getting quiet and raising my legs above my head to feel calm and rejuvenate myself. In yoga we call this, "Legs Up the Wall" pose. What happens is that blood rushes to the head and nourishes the brain, while feel-good hormones are released. It is a wonderful way to quickly feel peaceful and rested. I still rely on it to give me extra energy when I need it.

There is another way I keep my spiritual Self nourished. It involves rejigging my thoughts to be more heart-centered; in other words, more kind and nurturing. Reframing our thoughts to be more heart-centered and kind is a tried and true method of calming the brain and minimizing negative thoughts. I see it as the cornerstone of CBT.

My first experience with reframing occurred when I was five years old. I had watched an inappropriate program on TV and was terrified that pygmy voodoo dolls were under my bed. They had large spears and were trying to push them through my mattress. There were two warring tribes attacking each other and me. I was crying but no one came to my aid; perhaps there was an argument happening. So, after some time, I resolved the matter myself by having them become friends with each other and, of course, me. I must admit, this was very clever for a five-year-old to do! I believe that my guardian angels or spirit sent me the idea. Thank-you.

Another, more recent, example of reframing thoughts relates to the yoga classes I teach. Although I knew better, I would still sometimes fall into the trap of believing that if I had a full class, it meant that I was a good teacher. The problem with this thinking was that if only one or two people showed up on any given day, it meant that I was a bad teacher. Feeling like a bad teacher sapped whatever energy I had left. It was already a huge effort for this introvert to step up and teach. Not only was there a confidence factor, but, with my perfectionist tendencies, I would put a lot of effort into every class. It hardly seemed worth it if no one was going to show up.

My thinking had to change if I was to going to continue teaching. It is always impossible to predict how many students will attend a class, there are too many variables: holidays, finances, schedules, and so on. So, I reframed how I thought about my small classes; I began to think of them in terms of my own education. They became an opportunity for me to really hone my craft and enrich my teaching experience while helping my students to connect with Spirit in new ways. There is both a physical and a spiritual aspect to yoga, which helps us to get in touch with our bodies through physical movement and with our spirit through rest.

When I had a small class, I would draw on the advice in my collection of self-help books and read out passages that I had found meaningful in my life. Unbeknownst to the few students who had gathered, as time went on, I would test new approaches and try out more profound readings on them before the start of each class. Sometimes, when my beautiful yogis were getting centered and grounded, I would elaborate on the reading and give examples of how the principles it contained applied in the real world. After all, I thought that if it had helped me, maybe it could benefit them as well. A relaxed state is a receptive state. In my experience, a completely relaxed state promotes better insight and increased awareness. My intention was to encourage my students to pay more attention to the mind/body connection at a time when they were relaxed, open to Spirit, and therefore especially receptive. I know it was a little sneaky of me but I wanted to help raise their awareness and give them additional tools to improve their lives. It was also a way to build more community among all of those present. When we connect our bodies and minds in a peaceful way we feel safe to connect to others as well. I know that I certainly felt greater connection with my class, which was something of a breakthrough for me.

Community is another way to talk about human connection. It was around this time that I realized that, although spending time alone and getting quiet were important for connecting with Spirit, being part of a community also helps me to feel close to my spirit. In yoga we call it creating Sanga. As it turns out, the work I was doing with my smaller classes was not the first time that I had engaged in community building. I had been bringing people together for a very long time, albeit in other ways. I had always sought to create the connection and closeness that I craved for myself, but from a safe distance. It was a way to have a relationship with others and not feel so alone, without risking too much. It also helped to stave off depression, which occurs when we are socially isolated.

When I was only 18 years old, I started a baseball team at work. We were a group of like-minded people who wanted to win games and socialize afterwards. Years later, I was bringing people together for charity events. I once organized a yoga-thon at a local YM-YWCA where we raised money for at-risk youth. Again, we were a group of like-minded individuals coming together.

On another occasion, I joined a team of women who went into the community to connect with seventh and eighth grade girls. It was fun, exciting, and meaningful.

We spoke about our experience in terms of mental health, self-image, future goals, and vocations. Perhaps I was giving my younger Self the positive attention it had never received. I also helped to organize a luncheon for International Women's Day that offered free tickets to women who could not afford the fee. Then, came a very big event. I approached a local mental health agency about bringing PTSD awareness to first responders and high stress workers, such as teachers, child welfare workers, justice, medical, corrections, and family violence workers. It spawned a 5-year relationship with the agency and some wonderful symposiums. I see now how I was the one who benefitted the most from my community work. It was a way to heal myself.

Of course, yoga and the yoga community have been a constant healing for me in so many ways. I find yoga classes to be a community of very like-minded souls. I attend and continue to teach yoga classes, so my healing can continue. Whenever my husband and I are travelling we look for a yoga class and wherever we are, there is an instant connection that makes us feel welcome. We feel part of a larger movement and connected to each other through spirit. I have always thought that yoga was a component of a larger social justice movement, the peace movement.

I was a bit young to fully grasp the meaning of the peace movement in the 60s and 70s. I was very attracted to it, but couldn't participate in peace marches or demonstrations. I am sure, however, that my future Self knew that I would eventually engage in peace and non-violence activities. For me, that is yoga. Yoga is about peaceful connection with Self and others. I have also been very passionate about eliminating family violence —another kind of peace movement.

I thought that connecting with my spirit would be a mostly solitary journey; but perhaps, the key is to find a balance between going within and reaching out. Time we spend with others who are positive is so important. It helps us to live successfully in our busy, western society filled with negativity and mindless distractions. But being still and reflective is also important. When I spend some quiet introspective time on my own, analyzing how I feel and how I can be more positive, I can better navigate what is happening outside of myself. As I said, I can't control events but I can choose how to react to them. I like the idea of living mindfully and in balance; it helps me to make decisions with both my heart and my mind.

Speaking of being calm and mindful reminds me of a valuable lesson I learned from leading a men's domestic violence program I facilitated as a social worker. We talked about slowing down, trying to remain calm, and not over-reacting to our partners. The lesson was that by slowing down we could think rationally again and, if irritated, give our partners the benefit of the doubt. It was also easier to get and stay more positive.

Being calm gives us time to question whether what we are feeling and thinking matches the situation. Are we being proportional or are we engaging in one of the major "thinking distortions," such as catastrophizing and over personalizing? Those of us with loaded histories, often overreact in tense interactions with our partners. It may not seem like it, but that is a fear response, a sign of insecurity and feeling threatened. It is difficult to calm our fear once it is triggered, but if we slow down and connect with our thoughts and feelings, we can take full control and choose how to move forward. This is mindfulness at its best.

Fast Track Your Healing:

Getting Quiet

It is so important to find a morning or evening practice that helps to quiet your mind. Consistency is more important than total time spent being still. Here are some tips that I have found helpful:

Each morning, sit quietly for 10 minutes with your eyes closed, anywhere you feel comfortable like your bedroom, kitchen, or outside if possible.

If you are more comfortable with a moving meditation, you can walk mindfully, garden or fish in a quiet area, knit, gaze into a fire, or practice yoga alone.

To boost feelings of well-being, finish your quiet time with positive thoughts.

Knowing how to calm down comes in handy when feeling physically or emotionally threatened. If fear is activated, it is important to reduce your it as soon as possible.

Yoga: Doing yoga poses slowly and mindfully opens me up to new experiences because I feel safe to go forward and take small risks.

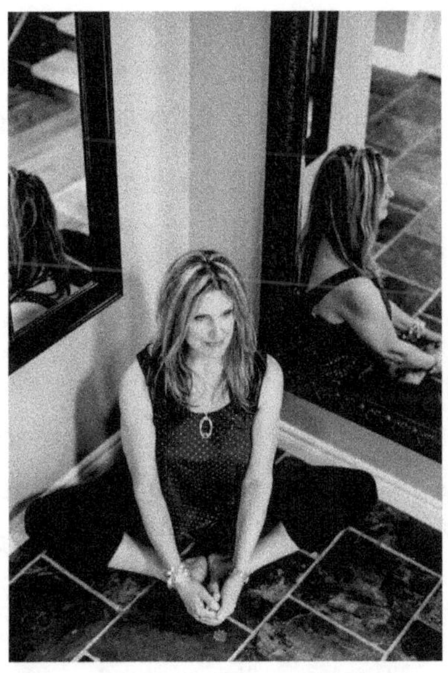

Meditation: Helped me to receive wisdom and inspiration from within, as well as accept myself. One day, during my morning stillness practice, I finally accepted that doing front-line social work was difficult. It affected my sense of safety and well-being, and does to this day. I asked myself if it was time to do less front-line work? The answer came back, yes. I put a plan in place to cut-back my hours drastically.

Chapter 10:

Feeling Safe

> *If you want to be happy, practice compassion.*
> *If you want to be happy, practice compassion.*
>
> **- Dalai Lama -**

Yoga Wisdom/Tool:

Trying to remain positive and giving people, including ourselves, the benefit of the doubt, contributes to having peace of mind and calm in our lives. We feel safer going about our business. There are so many benefits to having loving, heart centered thoughts or at the very least neutral ones. If I view the world and people in it as peaceful and safe to be around, I behave in the same way.

Are positive thinking, visualization, and re-framing with compassion really all that healing?

Over the years, I have developed some powerful coping strategies. Given my penchant for seeing the glass half-empty, it was imperative that I begin to feel safe and trust that my life was proceeding safely. I have learned that this can be difficult to achieve when our brains are on constant alert for potential danger.

Experiencing trauma of any kind can make a part of our brain, the amygdala, become over-active to say the least. Any hint of danger can send our sympathetic nervous systems into full action. In my case, this is especially bothersome when I am getting up at 2:00 am in the morning to go to the bathroom. Spoiler alert: I was blessed with an over-active bladder. Too much information I know.

As I get older, I have to go more often. What used to be a once a night occurrence, now happens two, three, even four times every night. With these numbers, the likelihood of me thinking about a negative incident that occurred that day or second-guessing some decision I have made, is high. This is especially true when I have had back to back clients. When that happens, I don't get enough time in between to process the session, to think of ways to better assist my client, and assess how they are doing overall.

Finally, I came up with a technique for ending the sleepless nights of worrying and ruminating about the same thing over, and over, and over again after a trip to the bathroom. To counteract disturbing thoughts, I recite whatever mantra pops into my head. On route to the bathroom I mentally start saying things such as, "I am loveable, I am safe, I am capable, I am healthy." The latter one is a frequent thought, especially if I feel a cold coming on. I am still a people-pleaser and do not want to cancel client appointments or yoga classes.

I also use other techniques when I have trouble falling asleep. I rely on "old school" methods, such as counting backwards from 10 to 1, telling myself I will be asleep by the time I reach 1. Sometimes, I have to repeat the process several times. Other times, I visualize putting all my concerns and worries into a basket and handing them over to God, the Universe, my Higher Power. I remind myself to trust that the Universe is there for me, guiding me throughout my life to safety. If I am really having a hard time with my repetitive thoughts and insecurities, I remember Little Holly. She obviously is unsafe and needs some TLC.

During these sleepless moments and hours, I visualize holding Little Holly in my arms and rocking her to sleep. It is a powerful self-soother for me and I have recommended it to clients as well. I tell her that she is safe and does not have to worry any longer. I have her back and will not leave her in the rubble again. I tell her I love her.

I must admit that saying that I love myself is very healing. It is probably the most healing and nurturing thing I can do in terms of calming my mind and relaxing. I tell Little Holly I am happy she is being brave and meeting new people. Believe it or not, this helps me to move out of my safety zone in everyday life. I used to be very fearful of meeting new people because I thought they would judge me. My soothing self-talk to Little Holly allows me to gently nudge past my fear and begin to enjoy meeting new people.

Talking to Little Holly allows me to separate myself from my fear. It allows me to take control and settle it down. I am no longer relating only to my fear-based self, I am accessing my parasympathetic nervous system and calming down. Self-talk is essential to accessing this part of me. If I am feeling lonely, unloved, or underappreciated, I tell Little Holly that "you are loved and loveable." I am opening up a part of myself that leads to an infinite source of wisdom and love. Is this my soul? Is this my luminous Self coming to the rescue? When I tap into this part of myself I access pure love. I highly recommend finding a mantra that resonates deeply with you. I also find that if, during the process, I also happen to remember another time when I needed positive and soothing self-talk, I can use my mantra to not only feel safe in the moment, but to apply it to the other past situation. It's as if a double healing and calming is taking place.

Another very powerful coping strategy I use to feel safe is reframing with compassion. Although it is not always possible, this strategy is most effective when used in the moment, when something upsetting is happening; when a situation has gone awry in some way and has become unpleasant. Having compassion for the other person makes their gestures or words appear less threatening.

I experienced just such a situation while writing this chapter. We were having work done on the house and the person doing it was someone that we had had issues with before. There had been problems with finishing work on time and to plan in the past, but we decided to give them a second chance. On the previous occasion, I had to dig deep and muster up some compassion for this person. Well, it seemed that the Universe wanted me to do it again. It was like a test of my coping strategy.

As I lay in bed that night, my anger and dissatisfaction were keeping me wide awake. After tossing and turning, I tried to distract myself with other thoughts. It didn't work. The feeling of persecution and taking it personally kept me super alert. My ego was in full control and fear started to set in. I finally remembered what had worked the last time and started sending compassion to this person. I thought, "It must be difficult for you at times and I am sure life is not always easy or fun." I thought that perhaps there was fear and maybe past trauma that were interfering in this person's life and preventing them from leading a happy, healthy life. I also thought that there were some medical issues that this person was struggling with, which only added to the problem.

I considered how difficult it was for me at times to feel positive and how even after a great deal of self-development work, I still tended to see the glass as half-empty. I chose to learn a lesson from our encounters and let the lesson play out. I also remembered that the

Universe had a grand plan for everyone that was far better and more loving than I could come up with myself. Today, I still have to regularly remind myself what I am grateful for in life, and how blessed I am, in order to feel more hopeful, and safe. I told myself that this person was on a journey just like I was, and that our paths had crossed for a reason.

I felt better and finally fell asleep after trusting that I would be safe. The next day, during my morning prayer and meditation time, I asked for guidance in writing this chapter and this situation came to mind. I recalled that I always remind my clients that we have choices in life: do we react in a way that makes us proud? Do we react in a way that gives us peace of mind? We do have the power, in these instances, to choose between positive, loving, or neutral thoughts about a situation, or to stay with the negative, unloving ones.

I took the suggestion that I give my clients. Instead of thinking that this person was out to get me and was judging me in some way, I chose to think in a loving manner; this person was not seeking revenge or persecuting me. I chose to see this person in a more light-filled manner. I chose to see this person's luminous Self. As I relaxed, I was once again reminded that peaceful thoughts equal a peaceful body, and vice-versa. As a result, I was able to interact with him in a pleasant way and feel safe as he finished his work.

The need for safety has been a recurring theme throughout my life. I learned so many beneficial lessons while working in the family violence field, I wonder if perhaps being a witness to violence as a child was a gift, of sorts, an opportunity to learn how to consciously induce feelings of safety in stressful situations. In the domestic violence program, we discussed slowing down, giving our partners the benefit of the doubt, not thinking we are being victimized in some way by them. I benefitted every time I heard these words of wisdom. Wisdom which allows for more peace of mind, more tools, and strategies I can use to feel safe and loving towards others.

The only difference between men and women who hurt their partners and those who do not, are how well they manage their thoughts and emotions. Again, peaceful thoughts and emotions, produce peaceful behaviour and vice-versa. Compassion produces peace as well.

Even if we can't forgive those who have harmed us, at the very least we can try to wish them well. This intention helps our brain turn thoughts of anger and fear into less emotionally charged ones; it can lead to more neutral thoughts or even, perhaps, thoughts of forgiveness.

Heart-centered thoughts activate the relaxation response, which calms us down. Today I try to be guided by the knowledge that I can always learn to manage and improve upon my reactions and my mental health each day, each moment. This gives me hope.

Fast Track Your Healing:

Positive Affirmations and Self-Talk for feeling Safe.

What we think, we become. My favourite manta is, "I am safe, people are safe, the world is safe."

Start your day by listing who and what you are grateful for along with some positive affirmations, which are also powerful change agents. Your affirmations don't have to be "pie in the sky", but they should be positive and hopeful.

If you add positive visualizations in anticipation of your day's activities, you'll switch on a powerful mechanism in your brain. Elite athletes know the benefit of going over their game or performance in advance of the event. They know that their brain will recall the visualization and try to make it happen in the real world. You can do the same thing.

Also consider using kind and positive self-talk after disappointments to increase your mental well-being. *Love always moves us forward.*

Yoga: Every time I get on my yoga mat, I am grateful and quietly bless myself and the other yogis in class. I also do this before and after teaching a class. In essence, I am sending out love and by doing so releasing "feel good" hormones like Oxytocin, Serotonin, and Dopamine.

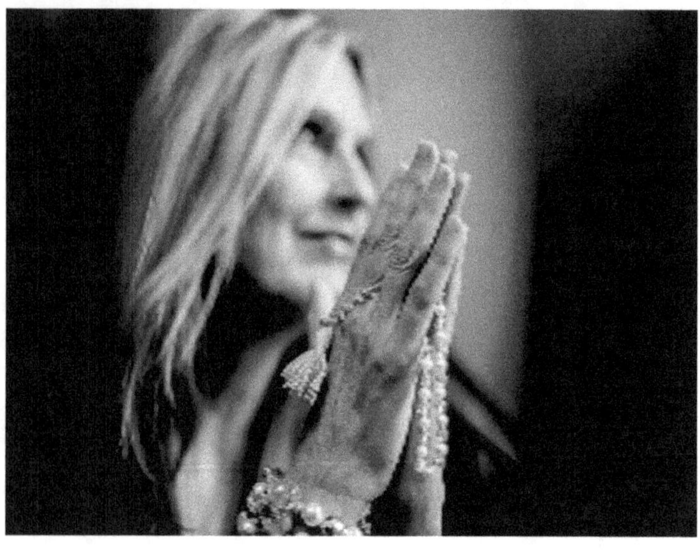

Yoga Pose: Blessing our enemies sends good energy to them, ourselves and into the Universe. The power of prayer has been researched and there is evidence that people who are being prayed for helps to accelerate their healing process. I bless my clients before each therapy session.

Chapter 11:

Taking Responsibility

Yoga Wisdom:

I listen for messages my body is sending me about people, places, and the food I eat.

Do we choose our experiences in order to learn?

After achieving some degree of serenity, I started asking some big questions about life. This tends to only happen once we have met the basic needs of safety and security. If we thought that the challenges we encounter in life happened to teach us how to be more loving and peaceful, would we be less resistant to them? Some New Agers believe that we choose our own life lessons including our parents, birthplace, and position in life. The more difficult the circumstances, the more we can advance in our journey towards total acceptance and love.

Perhaps, if we knew that there was a lesson to take away from every situation, we would be more likely to ask ourselves, "What was my lesson here?" Or, "How could have I reacted differently?" Perhaps we would take more responsibility for our side of the story. Knowing that we might have chosen this lesson, would we be less reactive and spend more time on understanding what we needed to learn? I know this can be a difficult concept to accept, especially for victims of violence, but looking for the lesson might have an empowering effect.

The survivors of even the most horrific events, who are able to accept their loss and move on with their lives, are often the ones who have found meaning in, or learned from, their experience. Lessons range widely, some are big, some are small, some are obvious, and some are more subtle. For example, some people learn, not only to accept help, but that they are loveable and worthy of that help. Others learn to stop worrying about the future, getting stuck in the past, or staying so busy that they don't notice what is happening here and now. They learn, instead, to focus on what is important now, like their child's birthday, which they may have missed in the past because they were so distracted. Still, others might discover that the image they cling so hard to, the one they want to project to the world in an effort to be liked or accepted, is not worth the worry and exhaustion. I can speak on that one from first-hand experience; it is impossible to control what others think about you or anything else.

It might be hard to believe, but some people feel *fortunate* for having experienced misfortune because they now feel more alive than ever. They have learned to totally accept themselves and their situation. Instead of caring about what others think, they now ask themselves what they really want. They check in with themselves and live a more authentic life. They choose to be themselves because, in that moment, they finally accept that they have enough, are doing enough, and are enough. The alternative would have been to stay miserable, which is no way to live.

Those who choose to learn from their experiences and fully accept themselves don't waste time worrying about whether they are enough or whether people like them or not. They understand that everything good and bad is transient, including their thoughts and feelings. In a sense, they practice a form of extreme mindfulness and true positive thinking. It's not that they don't feel sadness and anger but they know that their uncomfortable feelings will pass, which gives them a great deal of resiliency. They are able to sit with their feelings and accept what comes up. They are able to accept everything that happens in life, both pleasant and unpleasant because they are glad to be alive and have learned the value of the moment. They understand that to live fully is to accept the good, the bad, and the ugly and still see the beauty in the world.

Is it unrealistic to think that mindfulness, being in the moment, and reframing our thoughts can become second nature? That we can retrain our minds to come back to the moment, to our breath? That we can avoid being hi-jacked by our amygdala because we have learned effective coping strategies to deal with our anxiety, terror, and fear? The answer is, no. There are many techniques and practices available to us for overcoming our past and moving beyond our fears; I've described a number of them in this book already.

The key is to take responsibility. Responsibility for our self-talk, being mindful, getting what we want, our relationships, for how we build community, and for our health.

Our self-talk could go something like this, "Oh my friend, Fear, is back. What is it trying to teach me this time?" Then we could go through a process of inquiry to identify what we can and can't control. We would take responsibility for what we *can* control and make a conscious decision not to worry about what we can't. We could breathe into and consciously relax whatever is tightening up—neck, jaw, shoulders. Then when we are feeling more centered, we could consider what the best way would be to take care of ourselves in this situation. Now, when I experience anxiety or grief, for example, I try to bless myself and everyone else who feels the same way. I visualize enveloping all of us in love and light. It is good food for my Soul.

I associate mindfulness with responsibility because it is a choice. A mature choice. When we are mindful, not only can we avoid being overwhelmed by life's challenges, as discussed above but we can also live more consciously. We can be sensitive to the clues we receive; large or small. When I am being mindful, when I am not sure what my next step should be, I stay open to the possibilities even in casual, everyday situations. Inspiration can come from anywhere, in the music that happens to be playing on the radio when I'm driving or in idle chitchat with my husband and friends. For example, I remember when two friends of mine asked if the downstairs of my house was designed specifically to teach yoga. It was, although I hadn't used it for that purpose. But that was my cue to go back to teaching. I no longer teach at home, but that got me back to doing what I love.

Everyone is responsible for choosing to do what they want, what they love; to own their life and step fully into it each moment. I love helping people relax and get in touch with their bodies and souls. I don't care what anyone wears, brand-name yoga wear, or old sweatpants; I don't do it because it is trendy or makes me look cool. My only requirement is that my students use a safe, non-slip mat with a good, grippy surface for their feet. Teaching yoga is a sacred profession and so is being a therapist. I am blessed to be both and in both cases I help people connect their mind and body; I help them become more resilient and improve their mental health. I love serving in this way and I choose to do what I love. I often suggest volunteering to clients and friends who don't yet have the education or experience to work in the field that brings them joy.

Finally, if we want to feel good, we must all take responsibility for our health and well-being. Our body and our intuition send us signals that guide us to make healthier choices. Years ago, although I didn't realize it at the time, I responded to both external and internal messages that I was receiving about my health and the food I was eating. I listened, and it really helped my body. In my early twenties I started reading articles on the dangers of sugar and red meat. One story in particular stood out for me, it talked about how much undigested meat remained in the intestine and bowel of the average person when they die. I reflected on my diet and remembered feeling very different after eating steak versus fish or chicken. I felt heavier with red meat and did not digest it very easily. The information contained in the articles seemed consistent with the signals I was receiving from my body; I stopped eating meat.

I also eliminated salt and cut-down drastically on sugar. Today, I know when I have indulged in too much sugar or salt. I pay the price. I feel sluggish, thirsty, bloated, and my eyes are puffy. Now, I read labels and try to eat fresh vegetables, fruit, nuts, and legumes. I eat salt and sugar sparingly. I truly believe that lessons come in all shapes and sizes and from a variety of sources, including and especially from our bodies. I remind myself that I am never too old to learn and choose more positive and loving ways to respond to the world. Eating healthy food is part of that response, it helps me achieve both balance and calm. My choice of nutrition feeds my body and my spirit.

Fast Track Your Healing:

Responsibility.

Take Responsibility for your health by reducing guilty pleasures and nourish your Soul

There is a huge difference between taking an extra piece of chocolate and habitually having too much of it. Substitute whatever ie: alcohol, gambling, engaging in risky sex, binge eating, taking illegal drugs, or over medicating with prescription drugs.

If you think you are overdoing it, chances are, you are! If someone you know well thinks you are over-indulging, chances are, you are! Please listen to them, they love you.

If you are keeping whatever you are doing secret, you have a problem!

Reduce or eliminate the following from your diet to see and feel instant results:

"White Sugar, White Salt, and White Flour = White Death", my friends tease me when I say that, but if you can reduce or eliminate any or all of the above you will feel better, sleep better, and look better. You will lose weight, gain mental clarity, and have fewer digestive problems.

Not to mention reduce the risk of diabetes, heart disease, and the chance of having a stroke.

Most importantly, eliminate negative self-talk.

Yoga: As I get older there are some postures I cannot do, or do as well as I used to. Sometimes I have to make adjustments. I accept and go forward gracefully with loving awareness—without my fear-based ego sailing the ship.

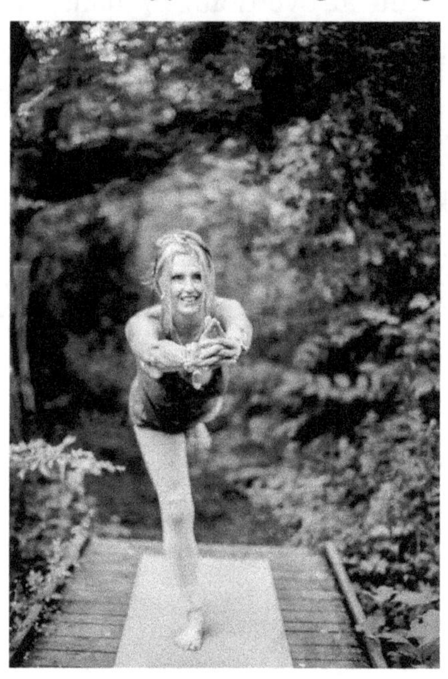

Yoga Pose: I cannot hold Warrior 3 or other more rigorous poses as long as I used to. I try and view the changes in a gentle and loving way. Getting down on my yoga mat as often as I can is more important than how long I hold each pose for.

Chapter 12

Vulnerability, Positive Thinking, and Trust

> *You can't heal what you can't feel!*
>
> *- John Bradshaw -*

Wisdom to live by at any age:

Don't feel silly if you are scared or intimidated when you enter situations where others wield total power and control over you. My usual mantra when I am feeling powerless is: "I am safe, I can do this. I am strong and brave." And, the next time will add "I trust this person has my best interests at heart" (unless they prove otherwise).

Vulnerability is good for me, why?

One day, during my morning quiet time, I asked to receive deeper lessons in my life. I had once heard Gabrielle Bernstein, one of my favourite authors, say something to this effect at a Hay House symposium and thought she was mad at the time. Now, I realize the wisdom in her request. Feeling very vulnerable and trusting that everything will work out can still be very difficult for me, so I thought this might be the lesson I needed to learn more fully.

The lesson came in two parts. The first began with a Facebook post about recognizing signs of breast cancer. As I stared at the pictures I remembered that I was late in booking a mammogram. I identified with some of the pictures and felt nervous. I booked an exam. As luck would have it, I called on a Friday and got an appointment on Monday. That left me with just two days to worry about what the mammogram would reveal.

I worked to remain calm and think positively over the weekend. More importantly, I tried to trust that whatever was meant to happen would happen, and I would deal with it. I got my mammogram and was a little paranoid when the technician had to take one picture a second time. I asked her if everything seemed ok and she said, "Nothing crazy is jumping out." Again, I tried to trust what she said. I went about my business and hoped I would not get a call the next day from my doctor. I thought I would get a call fairly soon if there was any concern. I didn't get the call and by Friday afternoon of the same week I called my doctor so I could relax.

When I called, I was informed, after some digging for my file, that the mammogram was normal. I was relieved to say the least. I took this episode as a lesson in trust and vulnerability. It was also a lesson in self-care. The breast screening organization is fairly good about sending out reminders, but, as I mentioned in the previous chapter, it is ultimately my responsibility to take care of my health.

Another lesson in vulnerability came by way of my teeth.

I mentioned earlier that Louise Hay associates tooth issues with decision-making. Well, I must admit that, coincidental or not, I was in the process of deciding what to do about the house we were living in at the time when this second lesson came about. This time my lesson was about expressing how vulnerable I felt and speaking my truth out loud to the person I was in conflict with. Speaking my truth was tied to trusting my truth.

Like most people, I don't enjoy going to the dentist. Being in a reclined position, not in control, and having someone's hands in my mouth is actually a very vulnerable position to be in. We all cope with it in our own way. I have to prepare myself each and every time I go to the dentist. I call on my best yogi breathing, mentally saying to myself that everything is going to be all right and that it will soon be over. To the staff, I must seem to be very high maintenance because I take in a rolled yoga towel to place at my low back, and I brush right before with toothpaste for sensitive teeth. I do this every time.

This time I was in to fill two, small cracks that had developed because of my nighttime tooth grinding. After a cleaning, the dentist had checked my teeth and informed me that I would need two fillings. I scheduled an appointment and arrived mentally prepared for the procedure the following week, my trusty yoga towel in tow. Because of previous root canal work, one tooth didn't require any anesthesia.

The other one needed to be frozen. The first filling only took seven minutes and I was glad we were moving along so fast. The second one, however, was more problematic.

I didn't know it at the time but the dentist had to scrape off a previous filling in order to fill the crack. This still does not make sense; however, because of this the procedure took about 35 minutes. It seemed like an eternity to me and when I asked for a break and inquired why this tooth was taking so long, I was informed of the removal of the existing filling. I was very upset that I had not been told about this procedure or how long it would take prior to booking the appointment. As the dentist resumed, it felt like I was drowning, there was too much water being piped into my mouth and the excess was running down my chin. I kept dabbing my mouth with a tissue and becoming more and more irritated. I was feeling that I was being treated like an object, with no control over what was happening to me.

As I was enduring the last part of the procedure, I decided that I wanted to talk to the dentist and I asked to see him after he was finished. I expressed my concerns and said that I was not given a proper explanation of what was going to take place. I argued that I had been unable to give the necessary informed consent because I hadn't known what to expect. They had just rushed through the explanation and failed to give me the information I needed to agree to the procedure. I also told him that I felt like an object. Even with my coping tools, when I get very upset it is difficult to remain calm and keep my voice from quivering and going higher and higher. I was very upset. Everyone was.

My dentist apologized and said that in the future he would make me fully aware of whatever I was getting done and how long it would take. I said thank you and asked them to let me know how long the cleaning would take the next time they left me a reminder message. They never reminded me. Perhaps there was another communication breakdown.

The problem with finding a new dentist, though, is that it doesn't matter who my dentist or hygienist is, I feel very vulnerable and uncomfortable every time.

After this incident I learned that it is my responsibility to ask questions if I feel that something is not being fully explained to me.

I also spent some time stewing over the cost of the visit, although my benefits would reimburse most of it. It was right after Christmas and I had paid with my credit card. What if it hadn't gone through? I told myself that the receptionist and the dentist didn't really care. That I was only a cash cow for them. I began to feel even more vulnerable and objectified.

But then, after some reflection, I realized that I was projecting my anger and feelings of helplessness onto them. I would have benefitted from more information, I have no doubt of that, but I was making them the villains and blaming them for how I felt when the intensity of my emotions had more to do with my history of trauma than the actual procedure.

I decided that the lesson for me, in this case, was to continue to take care of myself and to ask for help when I was feeling vulnerable; to explain when I felt anxious and afraid and needed help to get more comfortable.

I understand that feeling powerless is *my issue* and that I will have to live with it for the rest of my life; but asking for assistance will help calm my fears. I have no problem asking for assistance from a store clerk, but when I am in a powerless reclined position with sharp tools in my mouth, that's a whole other story. Still, by speaking to the dentist before a procedure, explaining that I need enough information to give informed consent, might convey how scary the experience is for me. I might feel more empowered and the dentist might be more understanding. One thing is for sure, Little Holly felt better after I stuck up for her and told the dentist how we felt. Here's to more truth telling!

I didn't fully make the connection between my anxiety at the dentist's office (or meeting a new massage therapist) and my history of cumulative trauma, until I sat down to write this chapter. It seems so clear to me now. I have been assaulted in the past, which added to my existing childhood trauma. It is the reason that I can easily feel objectified and taken advantage of by people. I feel even more helpless in the dentist's chair than my doctor's office. It is even more invasive, in some ways, with instruments in my mouth and up to two people working on me, physically dominating me. It puts me in a completely vulnerable position that has all of my brain's danger alarms going off at once.

Just writing about it triggers feelings of helplessness and anger. I wonder if the dentist and other professionals in the room realize just how difficult it is for some people to show up for their appointments. So, for all the women and men who feel like I do, who don't always receive the compassion and understanding they need to feel safe, I feel your pain. You are not alone.

Fast Track Your Healing:

When feeling vulnerable

If we think mindfully and with an open heart, we can always come up with people/places/things that we are grateful for. It helps us feel less alone and vulnerable, especially when going into scary situations.

Try and spend a few moments every morning and evening taking in and naming all of your blessings. It will help you to trust your path thus far, and going forward. It will also remind you that there is an abundant amount of goodness in the world. You are safe!

Give yourself a pat on the back when you have put your best effort into something, were the bigger person, or said a kind word in a difficult situation. You rock!

Yoga: I am in full control of my body and this makes me feel safe and empowered. I listen and proceed with kindness and love. I am beginning to feel safe more often than not, and hold more gentle poses longer, like the ones found in Yin yoga.

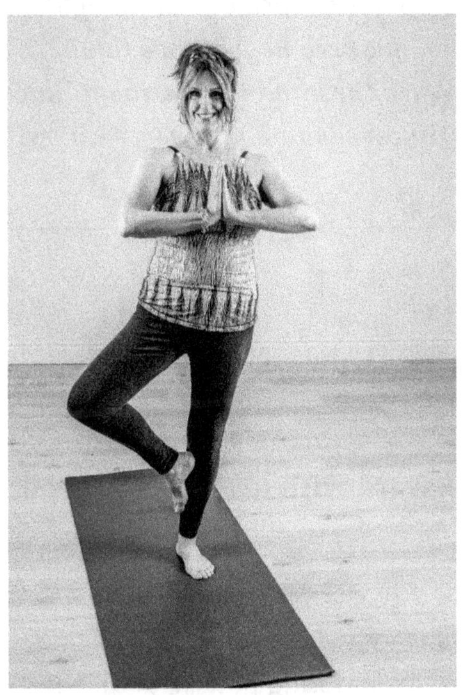

Yoga Pose: Tree pose helps to increase strength, balance and coordination. It helps us to focus inwardly and feel how our body is responding to the pose. It also helps us to stand in our truth!

Chapter 13:

Love, Fear, and Positive Intent

We are shaped by our thoughts,
we become what we think.
When the mind is pure, joy follows
like a shadow that never leaves.

- Buddha -

Yoga Wisdom:

Be in the moment; be fully in your body. Enjoy the sweetness!

Going forward with love, fear, and positive intent:

Life is like a river that sometimes flows quickly and sometimes slowly. It is not a straight line to serenity; it follows a meandering path with unexpected curves and switchbacks.

I wrote this book for two reasons. First, I wanted to help others by sharing my experience with finding some peace and serenity in my life. I love helping people, and this seemed like an exciting opportunity to do so.

Second, I wanted to provide some suggestions that would help people increase both their self-acceptance and their feelings of safety after experiencing trauma. I wanted to show how they could become their own loving therapist by making and holding space and honouring themselves. It might surprise you to hear this from me, but I have found that peace and serenity cannot be achieved by practising yoga alone. I wish it were that easy. Don't get me wrong yoga is very important. It helps us to get quiet and still, but it doesn't give us practical tips or techniques for dealing with feelings and the constant "go-to" thoughts that come up under stress. For me, CBT has been the best way to track, accept, and change my fear-based, critical self-talk.

I have found that acceptance, trying to be positive, and having loving thoughts is the best way to retain the calmness I feel after leaving the yoga studio. I used to have this wonderful, peaceful feeling for about five minutes after a class until I reached my car. Then, my old reality would take hold and all that good feeling would be lost. I could not have healed myself from the scary thoughts that I terrorized myself with, without the powerful help of CBT. I need both yoga and CBT to monitor how I am thinking, feeling, and reacting, but the latter is more effective for handling situations in the moment throughout the day.

Like many people, I wanted healing to take place right away, but there's no such thing as a quick fix. As another 12-Step saying goes, "It has taken years for you to get here, so it is going to take as long as it takes getting better." I spent years worrying about the opinion of others and believing that I was not worthy of happiness and joy. It will take time for me to learn how to think and feel differently. That's how it works, it takes time to change and develop new habits, but the place to start is with our thoughts, that's where real change happens.

Our mind and body are connected to each other but the mind is the chief executive officer. I used to read two or three self-help books every week but it was very frustrating because I wasn't getting any results for my efforts. I was sure that there must be something else wrong with me. I was following all of the steps and advice and still showing no improvement. The truth is that the processes contained in the self-help books would only feed my perfectionism and my need for instant results; if I wasn't getting results there was obviously something else wrong with me. Right? Wrong.

Thankfully, my degree in Philosophy provided some useful insight. My buddy, Socrates, once said, "An unexamined life is not worth living," which dove-tails nicely with Buddhist and Cognitive Behavioural thought. I needed to pay more attention to my thoughts and how they affected both my mood and, ultimately, my actions. If I was having a bad hair day, perhaps I should consider what I had been thinking when I got out of bed and started getting ready for the day. What were my thoughts when I first looked in the mirror? Was my hair all that different from yesterday? Or were my thoughts darker and more unaccepting? Less loving?

I had monitored my thoughts and reflected on my subsequent actions for years, but one day an event really drove home the importance of the process in my life. I was co-facilitating a group for men who had sexually offended, which is difficult work. The lead facilitator asked the men to monitor and journal their thoughts to identify any that might put them at risk of acting out sexually and offending. How did these thoughts make them feel and act? In effect, they were micromanaging their actions by paying strict attention to their thoughts. They were also asked to do something that made them happy or brought them joy; something healthy. I was amazed at the simple activities they did to feel good; small but positive actions that made a world of difference to their outlook and well-being.

I was also surprised at the progress that they made during the 12-week program. For many, it was the first time that anyone had asked them to do something that brought them happiness, that made them feel good about themselves. I started asking myself the same questions. What had I done that week to bring me joy? What simple, small actions had I taken? I had no answer. Even after working on my personal growth for many years I still didn't have a clear answer to this question. I started paying even more attention and being more mindful of my thoughts and actions, and how they left me feeling. That's when I realized, for the first time, that how I felt was totally within *my* control. I decided to give myself permission to bring joy into my life.

My happiness was not controlled by others, as I had thought for most of my life. It was under my control. I could just ask myself what I wanted, what next step would bring me joy. What did I want to eat? Whom did I want to connect with? How could I accept myself more readily in this moment? How could I be more loving with others and myself? How should I choose to react to situations like the one at the dentist's described in the last chapter? Should I choose to forgive or hang on to a grudge? Which option made me feel more empowered and in control?

I chose to forgive the dentist and for me this was empowering. Again, just because I forgive someone doesn't mean we have to be best friends. I don't even have to like them. I can choose to continue with the relationship or, if trust has been broken, I can choose to move on. When it comes to how I react, the choice is mine. The decision is mine alone. We all have lessons to learn. Perhaps I was meant to be a lesson in my *dentist's* journey. As long as I am not being hurt by this individual, I have options. If I am unsafe, I need to leave the situation and the person as soon as possible.

I have found that the only way I can truly forgive someone and move forward in whatever manner I choose is to *not* take the situation personally. I try to see that the other person was doing the best they could at the time and did not mean to hurt my family or me, no more than I have when I have hurt others in the past.

We are all doing the best we can. Some people are very aware, others less so, and some are just asleep at the wheel when it comes to any awareness of how their actions impact others. But it isn't really about them; it is about how you choose to react to them. Personalizing, being offended, staying hurt are disempowering responses to have. I don't want to live there, do you? It is more productive to ask, "What is this situation triggering within *me*?" Am I seeing reality correctly? If I'm feeling unsafe, what mantra is needed? "I am safe, brave, and trust everything will work out."

Fast Track Your Healing

Lighten Up, You are Human, You Make Mistakes

We all need to take a break from self-reflection and introspection. Sometimes we need to have fun. Be silly. I know I do. I ask Little Holly what she really would like to do. She is still pretty serious and could use a little fun once in a while.

Or, if you need a boost you can make a quick mental list of everything you are grateful for in your life, how much abundance there is all around you, who you have in your life. This could be your neighbour, the store clerk you see every day, or a distant relative. In doing so you will be releasing all feel-good hormones and your mood will improve. Thoughts and feelings go hand in hand.

Embrace your beautiful, messy life. We are not robots!

If you are taking yourself too seriously, try intentionally making a mistake to test your self-talk and choose to laugh at yourself. Be supportive, nurturing, and lead from the heart.

Try taking life less seriously, indulge is some silliness and bad puns. Here, I'll go first:

Why was the woman angry after a yoga class? *She was bent out of shape.*

Someone said they could not do yoga because *it was a stretch for them.*

Yoga wisdom: Finding a yoga teacher and class where you feel safe and welcome is very important. Thanks to my yoga teachers, past, present and future.

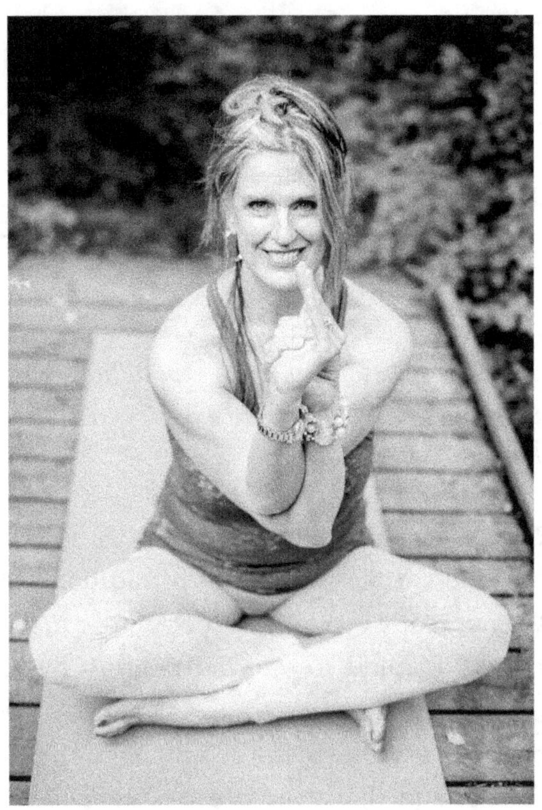

Yoga tip: I try to ask myself, "How can I be more loving in this pose?"

Chapter 14

Yoga and getting to the Good Stuff

> *Yoga is the journey of the self,*
> *through the self,*
> *and to the self.*
>
> *- Bhagavad Gita -*

Yoga Wisdom:

Only when we release all outside expectations of what we think we should be, do we get to our essential Self. Full of love, light, and wisdom.

I am sure everyone will agree that yoga is extremely popular today. Yoga is an eastern tradition but since the 60s it has really increased in popularity in the West. It has been adapted to varying degrees by western yogis to suit western tastes, in an effort to provide options for everyone. Some would argue that doing yoga is cool and that therefore we are cool if we do yoga. When I start thinking this way, which has happened before, I know my ego is involved. Ego is fear-based and always grasping for more, which is not conducive to having the internal peace and equanimity that yoga can give us.

Yoga provides numerous benefits, such as stress reduction, lower blood pressure, organ detox, mental clarity, increased focus and concentration, emotional balance, among others. By consistently getting on our mats and combining breath with movement, we not only transform our body but also our mind, from the inside out.

I first came to yoga in the 80s when Jane Fonda (I love you Jane) was telling us to "feel the burn" and soldier on. Like everyone else, I was into aerobics and wearing legwarmers that did little to relieve the leg cramps as we powered through the class. My ego was in full force clamoring for me to buy color coordinated workout apparel that matched my sneakers. Back then, like today, the active wear industry competed for our dollars. Now, I totally get why Indian yogis and yoginis all wear the same outfits: plain white robes or tunics and comfortable pants. It is easier to keep the Ego in check when everyone isn't competing to be the best-dressed, trendiest person in the room. It is hard enough to avoid getting caught up in doing yoga the "right" way and keeping up with the other students, without worrying about making a fashion statement too.

When I returned to yoga, after getting sober, my attitudes had changed, but it still took a while for that ego to quiet down. In order to penetrate to my inner layers, where the good stuff is, I had to shut out as much of the outside world as I could while staying present for the class and the instructor. And, of course, I avoided the mirrors; still judging myself, especially my body.

I tried not to look around to see what others were doing. Instead, I checked in with my body to see what felt right. I made sure that my joints were properly stacked for the pose and that I felt secure. I took my time when the instructor asked us to go deeper into a pose. My initial tendency had been to immediately oblige the request, but, after attending several classes, I learned to move at my own pace. I would even wave an instructor off if they wanted to help me go deeper and I didn't feel up to it.

I learned not to allow myself to be "bossed around" by well-intentioned teachers, or to feel shame for not keeping up with the class. I just chose not to worry about keeping up with the others and it felt wonderful. I was learning to accept myself where I was at and it was empowering.

I really had to get over my ego when I became a yoga teacher. I had come to the very sensible conclusion that I didn't have to be the best in the class to be a teacher, but to do that I had to set aside my ego and my fear of judgment. I chose to accept that I am human, that I have physical issues and limitations, but that I could still be a good teacher. I hope that I can inspire others with this story. It is all about accepting yourself. By eventually accepting myself, and my physical quirks, I was able to successfully overcome my fears, work through my doubts, and do what I loved.

Yoga helped to quiet my people-pleasing and perfectionist tendencies. But these were put to the test when, after I had been teaching for a few years, the Gentle Yoga classes I loved to teach were cancelled. They were replaced with hot yoga and some trendy class which entailed ropes and hammocks hanging from the ceiling. I was not interested in getting trained in either, and so was not needed.

My ego took a hit on several levels, but I sensed that I should keep touting the benefits of a gentle and mindful yoga practice even though I had to stop teaching for a few years because of the lack of interest. I did attend some of the more popular classes but knew that they were not for me. In fact, I incurred a number of injuries in hot yoga: I went too far into a pose when my muscles were relaxed and regretted it later as I walked out into the cold air, or I over stretched and had to take a few days off while my muscles recovered. Part of the problem was that it was difficult to keep my ego totally out of my practice as I tried to keep up. But it just wasn't what I needed. Please don't get me wrong, hot yoga can be very beneficial, but unfortunately my body was starting to slow down and was not as flexible.

Constantly checking in with myself, which I did during yoga classes, had the unintended benefit of developing into what would become a life-long practice of self-acceptance and kindness toward myself and others. Self-acceptance and kindness are where we find our perfect, higher Self. It is where we can make decisions and plans that are aligned with Love. This is the good stuff we get to as we go within and accept ourselves unconditionally; as we give ourselves loving encouragement, compassion and appreciation.

Everyone's yoga journey is different but, for me, after my ego relaxed, I found that the most healing poses were Child's pose and Bridge pose. I felt safe in Child's pose and empowered but not too exposed in Bridge pose. I was able to nurture myself in Child's pose and support myself in Bridge pose.

I was taught that there is a psychological component to each pose, in addition to its physical aspect. I felt strong and kind while in bridge pose as it opened my heart while connecting with my mind. They say that bridge pose creates a bridge between our head and heart. Both are needed to make decisions and go forward. Child's pose felt safe and I was completely protected. I could protect myself.

Over time, it didn't matter what I was wearing or how I was doing my pose in relation to other people. What mattered was that I was accepting myself. I was staying in the moment and not distracting myself with my ego driven thoughts. I was being with myself and it felt wonderful.

My negative self-talk, judgment, and second-guessing diminished greatly. I felt strong and at peace with myself. I felt joy. I had stripped away the criticism and shame and was left with acceptance of others and myself. I started to smile when leaving the yoga studio and I felt connected to the other yogis in the class. I was not alone; we were interconnected. This is the good stuff.

When I hear people say they are handling stress better, feeling better about themselves, or are more patient, I know that they are feeling the good stuff. The Gentle classes I teach now have just one purpose —peace. Unfortunately, there are still many people who don't appreciate a slower, mindful practice but it has its fans. I have found that retirees, artists, and musicians value the added benefits it brings. They seem to be more attuned to their inner world, more interested in creativity and contemplation. They understand that there is a place where they can connect with a force beyond themselves where they will find inspiration and peace, as well as physical and emotional healing.

I hope I have inspired you to go out and seek it.

Fast Track Your Healing

Accept, Be Still, Calm your mind through your breath

Find your unique way to meditate.

Then meditate, meditate, meditate.

Postscript

> *Acceptance looks like a passive state,*
> *but in reality*
> *it brings something entirely new into this world.*
> *That peace, a subtle energy vibration, is*
> *consciousness.*
>
> *- Eckhart Tolle -*

Yoga Wisdom:

Trust. You've got this!

Why am I taking two steps forward and three steps back? But, is it really back?

Throughout the book I have tried to weave together yoga and positive self-talk and sought to demonstrate how they can heal emotional wounds. Deep wounds are a result of having suffered some sort of trauma in our life. For me, having a history of trauma has been a blessing and curse. As an old Buddhist saying goes, "Could be good, could be bad." I don't talk about the exact nature of my trauma because I don't believe in re-traumatizing myself or anyone else. I don't believe in the value of re-hashing events in my life that have been terrifying, that I have felt ashamed about, or that have filled me with constant negative self-talk and guilt. I *do* believe in seeing the glass as half-full, so, as I move forward, I try to focus on the gifts I have received, on feeling empowered, and on loving. I manage symptoms by identifying feelings of fear, anxiety, and sadness, and knowing they will pass. I breathe through them.

I also don't need an official medical diagnosis of vicarious trauma or PTSD to know that I have suffered, and still suffer, from trauma. A recent, apparently innocuous event, really brought home just how deeply entrenched my feelings of being unsafe are and how much awareness and work are required for me to stay calm.

I wanted to switch to using non-toxic cleaning products and soaps in my home, so I contacted the distributor and spoke with a lovely representative. After placing the order, I realized that there had been a miscommunication. I found out that I would receive an automatic monthly shipment of my original order unless I continued to place orders each month. This made me mad. I felt that something was being imposed on me, as if I was being forced to buy. I felt unsafe and not in control. When I contacted the representative about the automatic shipment, she helped me cancel and get out of the system entirely. What a relief.

I happened to be doing some mirror work at the same time through Hay House and I believe the intense, personal connection with Little Holly made me feel safe enough to learn about and honour my fear on a deep level. As a result, I was able to address the source of my anxiety, the automatic shipment, and remove it in a healthy proactive way.

I asked myself why the automatic shipment incident bothered me so much. Why did I assume my representative did not have my best interests at heart even though she is a lovely, kind soul? What came back gave me huge insight into how my past trauma was coloring my response to everyday interactions. My trauma issues had surfaced in this instance, as they had in the dentist's office. I realized that even though I have overcome many challenges, I can still feel that people are out to get me, and that I am not being heard, which triggers other insecurities, fear, and anger. Most people are not out to get me, I understand that intellectually, but the feeling of victimization is still there.

Negative and fearful self-talk have been with me my entire life, the difference is that now I have effective tools for lowering the intensity of these feelings and shortening their lifespan. Living in a state of constant vigilance might seem like a curse, but I don't see it that way. For me it is a way to stay in touch with my feelings, in control of my reactions, and to learn to live mindfully.

It also makes me a good therapist and yoga teacher. Helping others to feel safe and calm is one of my greatest joys in life. My own experience with trauma helps me to provide a gentle and safe environment. If they didn't feel safe, my students and clients wouldn't feel they could gently stretch themselves, both literally and figuratively. They need to feel safe to try new poses, new behaviours, new ways of thinking about their life, and to take some risks.

If our purpose in life is to learn to be more loving, then our challenges are lessons sent from the Universe to help us get there. Did the Universe send me lessons in the shape of my dentist, my mammogram, and, yes, even a mix-up about automatic monthly shipments, to help me be more loving and at peace? Instead of looking at my recent panic attacks and feelings of being unsafe as steps backwards, I chose to "walk the talk" and look at them in a more positive light.

Perhaps, these situations are helping me to understand, accept, and love myself even more. Now, I feel that I can trust that I have the ability to get through whatever challenge comes my way, that my Higher Power is always with me and waiting for me to call upon her/him/it when I need help. I also know now, that I have to remember to be tender with Little Holly. Instead of shaming her about being immature and having ridiculous fears, I need to love her. I need to reassure her that everything will be okay.

Speaking of Little Holly, inner child work is very beneficial for both men and women to address the negative effects of self-criticism and fear. I have counselled many men who have tender little boys inside them who are waiting to be acknowledged and told everything will be okay. They need to hear that that they don't have to run away from their fears by drinking and drugging them away, or by getting angry.

My own inner child work began many years ago. Following the advice of Bradshaw and his remarkable work, I purchased a doll that reminded me of myself – if you guessed Holly Hobby you will have guessed correctly. I took her everywhere. She sat in the front seat of my car and worked alongside me during my sales rep days. It was a little weird at first, but it didn't take long for me to get used to having her at my side. The doll was a reminder that I was precious and needed to be loved, not to be abandoned. If I took care of her, she was also proof that I could keep myself safe. I mention this experience only to illustrate that there are many different techniques available to you to help move you toward recovery. Again, I suggest you find what works for you.

I believe that it was my intense inner child work that gave me the courage to leave my lucrative sales job and go back to school. I was terrified of leaving my job but I knew it was the next logical step for me to take. I owed it to my Self, and to Little Holly; she always wanted an education and it turned out to be the best thing I could have done. I was the first person in my family to get a university degree. I was very proud of myself and very thankful that my husband was on board with the idea.

Combining inner child and mirror work has helped me immensely to feel safer. When I look in the mirror now, I see something very different than I did when I was young. I remember staring at my eyes in the bathroom mirror when our parents were out for the evening; they had left my older brother in charge. I was very worried about my parents. I was worried they would not come home. I didn't feel safe and I started to cry. I looked deeply into my eyes and couldn't come up with any soothing words, I felt abandoned and alone. I am so glad that, now, when I look into my eyes, I am able to give myself the reassurance I need to feel safe, to trust that everything will work out the way it is supposed to.

In addition to all of the personal development and inner child work that I to do to manage my fears, I also try not to terrorize myself with morbid thoughts anymore, although I still do sometimes. It is a coping mechanism that I haven't yet been able to shake. I think I do it as a way of protecting myself from bad feelings.

If I think about the most distressing outcome possible, and really feel it in the moment, then I know that I can survive it when it really happens. For example, I have gone over what I would say at a loved one's funeral. It doesn't really make me feel better or that I could cope if someone close to me dies. Morbid thoughts only add to my gloomy and fearful state. It isn't good for me. Instead I would do better to remind myself that the glass is half-full and to enjoy every minute I have with my loved ones. I am working on it.

It is true that as you get older you appreciate who and what you have in your life more, a lot more. When I fall back on old fears of being judged or rejected, I fill myself with positive self-talk and how much I love being around people and enjoy the connection. I try to savor the moment by not rushing home immediately after having dinner with my family or friends, or lingering after a yoga class to chat.

Still, sometimes, our closest relationships can be very difficult to navigate as we try to remain present to what is happening and how we are feeling. We want the connection but we don't want to be triggered into an anxiety attack or some other fear response. That's why it is so important to have good tools to help us cope. If we stay aware and listen to our bodies, we can use techniques like positive self talk and breath work to remain calm and avoid an emotional crisis. Of course, a major part of being willing to risk a connection, to spend more time in the company of others implies a willingness to be vulnerable. It means allowing people to see who we really are and not getting upset if we don't click with everyone.

When you have experienced trauma, it can be difficult to know how to establish appropriate boundaries in your relationships.

I speak from experience when I say how difficult it is to engage with others sometimes, when you have spent an entire lifetime being unsure of what those boundaries should be. Most of the time, I was either too controlling or not controlling enough. My jobs have usually been positions of control, ranging from waitressing to being a probation and parole officer; and if you think that in addition to towering over you, your server doesn't have much power over your meal, think again.

For me, having appropriate boundaries now means allowing people to come in and out of my life in an easy, mentally healthy way. I try to be fluid and malleable. If I slide backwards, it is because I am feeling unsafe. I take it as a signal for me to slow down or re-think my position, which is a much more positive response than I would have had in the past. So, it is not really taking a step backwards but rather a test of my new awareness, one that confirms that I am on the right path and that my action plans and tools for happiness are working.

What does it really matter if I still can't nap in the afternoon? To date, I have not felt safe enough. Perhaps, one day I will be able to have a wonderful snooze, or not. Either way, I accept where I am and look forward to whatever the Universe has in store for me. I look forward to feeling even safer. To feeling more love and more peace. I know these feelings will continue to deepen as I continue my daily affirmation practice. I know they will materialize as I am affirming that they already have. Visualizing them in my life has already given me a greater sense of contentment, trust, acceptance, and connection. I know that the Universe has everyone's best interests at heart, including mine.

I believe that our dreams will come true, so I am dreaming bigger these days.

Namaste, my luminous, light-filled travellers.

Reach for the stars, my friends, you can touch them.

Recommended Reading

A Course in Miracles by Helen Schucman

Transforming the Pain: A Workbook on Vicarious Trauma by Karen W Saakvitne and Laurie Anne Pearlman

The Presentation of Self in Everyday Life by Erving Goff (authenticity and hiding our real selves)

You Can Heal Your Life by Louise Hay (mind/body connection and affirmations)

The Universe Loves You by Louise Hay and Robert Holden (mirror work)

Homecoming: Reclaiming and Championing Your Inner Child by John Bradshaw (inner child work)

A Return to Love by Marianne Williamson (forgiveness and much more.)

Man's Search for Meaning by Viktor Frankl (forgiveness and much more)

Embracing Ourselves by Hal and Sidra Stone (embracing your entire being)

The Dark Side of the Light Chasers by Debbie Ford (embracing your entire being)

Resilience: Powerful Practices for Bouncing Back from Disappointment, Difficulty and Even Disaster by Linda Graham (trauma/mind/resilience)

Synchronicity by Carl Jung (coincidences and synchronicity)

Daring Greatly: How the Courage to Be Vulnerable Transforms the Way We Live, Love, Parent and Lead by Brene' Brown (vulnerability/acceptance and resilience)

Light on Life: The Yoga Journey to Wholeness, Inner Peace, and Ultimate Freedom by B.K.S. Iyengar (yoga wisdom)

The Wisdom of Yoga: A Seeker's Guide to Extraordinary Living by Stephen Cope (yoga wisdom)

Conscious Femininity by Marion Woodman (honouring intuition/nurturing/feminine qualities)

Internal Family Systems Therapy by Richard K. Schwartz

Buddha Brain: The Practical Neuroscience of Happiness, Love and Wisdom by Rick Hanson

Second Hand Shock: Surviving and Overcoming Vicarious Trauma by Ellie Izzo and Vicki Carpel Miller

Bodhisattava Mind Audiobook by Pema Chodron

With So Much Gratitude....

Many people and coffee shops have helped me write this book. I first want to thank my book mentors, teachers, and therapists who guided me to safety many, many times in the past. My professors who allowed me to use my voice in my essays, which allowed me to grow, learn, and apply the theory they were teaching to my life. And, to my clients, yoga students, and everyone who has participated in the various groups I was a part of—you are brave and light-filled.

I am so grateful to my meditation and yoga teachers. You all helped me to go beyond the surface, so the authentic part of me could emerge. In addition, I received so much help from body practitioners over the years. Childhood trauma caused fear and emotional energy to remain stuck in my body and it needed to be released. I have used and continue to use massage, reflexology, and Traeger body work to heal. I thank my favourite and most challenging yoga postures for assisting in that healing.

Thanks to the team at Follow It Thru Publishing for the much needed hand-holding and support. Your suggestions were positive and kind. You are all amazing. And, to Laynie from Jono and Laynie Co. for the wonderful pictures.

I thank my family and friends. Without your love and support I would not be here today. You are always on my mind, even if there are miles between us. An extra special thanks to my childhood friends who have always accepted all of me. There were many times our friendship helped me to limp along just knowing you were there for me. My step-sons have been my teachers so many times without knowing it. Thank you, to both of you. I do believe our children are our greatest teachers. And to my beautiful and kind granddaughters; it is true that you can do no wrong in my eyes.

If people are assignments who help us grow more loving and kind, I have to thank my biggest teacher, my spouse who is the most loving and patient person I know. I can only hope I have shown you the same devotion and loyalty you have shown me. You cannot begin to know how important they have been to my journey and me.

Wishing you much Love and Light,

Holly. ॐ

About the Author

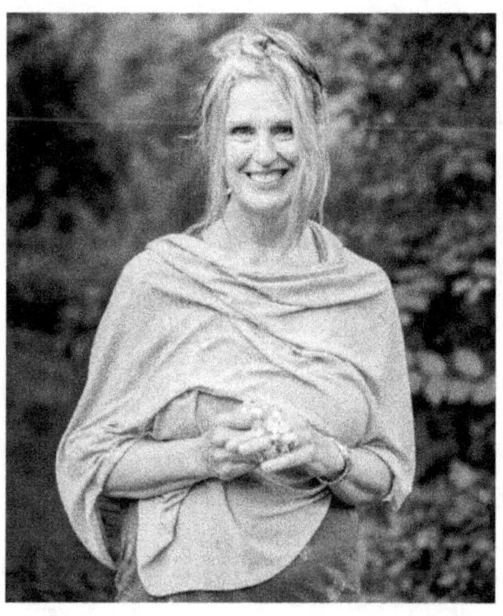

Holly McDonald is a life-long learner and engages in daily spiritual practices. She is a yoga teacher and therapist who helps her clients and students to make their mental health and well-being a priority. She firmly believes that transformation, peace, and resiliency are possible and that they are our birthright. Holly holds Master's Degrees in psychology and social work, as well as yoga certificates. Holly realizes that living with the effects of past trauma requires on-going awareness and positive self-talk to both navigate life in a healthy manner and live as peacefully as possible. She continues to practice yoga and mindfulness to ensure her life is happy and loving. Holly believes that compassion for Self comes first and that only then can it be offered freely and openly to others. She lives in a small lakeside community, or Sanga, in Ontario, Canada, with Ian, her beloved partner of many years.

https://www.hollymcdonald.org/